IT'S PROBABLY YOUR HORMONES

Dr Mary Ryan trained at Trinity College Dublin and obtained her MB BCH BAO MA MD MRCP in 1992. She completed her Specialist training in endocrinology. She is a regular contributor to the media, a senior lecturer at the University of Limerick and host of the *Empowering Women* podcast.

www.drmaryryan.com

IT'S PROBABLY YOUR HORMONES

From appetite to sleep,
periods to sex drive,
balance your hormones
to unlock better health

Dr Mary Ryan

QUERCUS

First published in Ireland by Gill Books in 2023

First published in Great Britain in 2023 by

QUERCUS

Quercus Editions Ltd
Carmelite House
50 Victoria Embankment
London EC4Y 0DZ

An Hachette UK company

A CIP catalogue record for this book is available from the British Library

TPB ISBN 978 1 52943 486 6
Ebook ISBN 978 1 52943 487 3

10 9 8 7 6 5 4 3 2 1

Illustrated by Derry Dillon
Designed by Typo•glyphix, Burton-on-Trent, DE14 3HE
Printed and bound in Great Britain by Clays Ltd, Elcograf S.p.A.

MIX
Paper | Supporting
responsible forestry
FSC® C104740

Papers used by Quercus are from well-managed forests and other
responsible sources.

*I would like to dedicate this book to mná na hÉireann
and all the women who have been so unnecessarily
misunderstood about their hormonal health.
I hope that this book can help them on their journey.*

*I also want to dedicate it to my three wonderful children,
Micheál, Seán and Úna; my parents, Seán and Úna;
and my siblings and friends.*

Contents

'The trick is in what one emphasises. We either make ourselves miserable or we make ourselves happy. The amount of work is the same.' – Carlos Castaneda

'If I am not good to myself, how can anyone else be good to me?' – Maya Angelou

Introduction

Hormones have taken me all over the country and all over the world. These tiny little receptors are responsible not only for millions of actions in the human body but for my entire career in medicine. Hormones are chemicals that produce and control every muscle and organ in the body. What fascinates me the most is how little we know about them but how hugely important they are to everything in health.

Hormones are our engine, our motivators and the essence of our being. They determine our sex, our emotions, our highs and our lows, how we wake up, how we sleep, when we eat, when we fall in love and who with. They give us happiness. They inform our cells about the steps to take in the body and make sure they all communicate with each other. Without hormones, our bodies could not function. Without the hormone ghrelin that controls hunger, we would not survive as it prompts us to eat and store up proteins, fats and carbohydrates.

Hormones give us the strength to fight, thanks to the hormone adrenaline produced by our adrenal glands. They are messengers that operate in a circadian rhythm and have a very controlled negative and positive feedback system which I believe is far more intricate than any computer or technology we have here on earth. Like all great systems, it needs to work in synchronisation, and when we overdo it, get ill or have severe hormone fluctuations, this has a knock-on effect on every other system in our body. When a single hormone is out of sync it can disrupt all other hormones.

Hormones dictate our daily rhythms, stabilise our immune system, keep our brain fit and regulate our appetite and core body temperature. They operate muscle and bone growth, the menstrual cycle, our feelings and our moods. The hormonal cycle is determined by supply and demand. Because the tiniest amount of a single hormone can have such an impact and because hormonal control loops are complex, the hormonal system is vulnerable to stress and sleep deprivation.

A holistic approach is key when we are examining hormonal imbalance. If we truly love ourselves we must understand our hormonal vortex, look after it, respect it and nourish it.

I have been fascinated by the hormonal system since I began my medical training as a student at Trinity College Dublin. I was lucky to be taught by incredible teachers and being a woman in medicine at that time brought a very different dynamic to my studies. There were very few female mentors in Trinity while I was there, apart from my wonderful anatomy teacher Professor Moira O'Brien and the obstetrician Professor Patricia Crowley. These brilliant minds were inspirational to me and shaped the doctor I was to become.

Introduction

When I first started, I was interested in cardiology and thought that was the area I would specialise in, but I was lucky to be assigned to the Adelaide and Meath Hospital where I worked as an intern for Dr John Barragry and Professor Gerald Tomkin, who were both endocrinologists. Like most people, I barely knew what endocrinology was at that time, but through their teaching and mentorship, I became fascinated by hormones and how they control absolutely everything.

Dr Barragry and Professor Tomkin taught me a holistic approach to medicine, which was maybe a little unusual at the time but is something that I have kept close to me in my practice ever since. They showed me how our hormones are interwoven with every system and taught me to treat the entire person as a whole. I loved this – I felt like I was a detective trying to tie the story together.

I can remember seeing patients and understanding for the first time that endocrinology is not straightforward medicine. It requires you to go behind the scenes, try to figure out what's going on and ask a lot of questions.

You have to look underneath to find the source of the problem. The key is to look at all the systems together and not just one system at a time (which is what you might do in different specialities). In endocrinology, it's the interplay between them all. For example, if a female patient comes to me with severe fatigue, I have to check that her periods are not too heavy and that they have not caused a hormonal imbalance, but I also have to check that her thyroid is normal and that all other systems are also working well, as hormones control them all.

I was fascinated by how tiny hormones work like medical messengers in the body and how without them the body would not function. I was also enthralled by how there was still so

3

much more to be learned in this area and that we were only in the foothills of everything we know now.

I was intrigued by how a tiny pea-sized gland – the pituitary gland – at the base of the nose could control a whole body. The positive and negative feedback system was so intricate, and I knew how much more I had to learn.

One of Dr Barragry and Professor Tomkin's key teachings, and one I carry with me to this day, was how important it is to take a good patient history. You cannot underestimate the importance of good listening skills and honest communication; understanding that is a must for every future doctor.

What your patient tells you and how you listen can give you so much information about what's going on. Examinations and the appropriate tests are very important, but you don't know what you're looking for if you don't listen to what you're being told by your patient and ask them the right questions. Your communication skills are key to getting the correct diagnosis.

While I was training with Professor Tomkin, I began to see how much of an impact hormones have on women's health in particular. The thyroid is a huge issue all round, but very common in women in particular and especially relevant for fertility. We came across a patient who had gone through about eight rounds of in vitro fertilisation (IVF), which was physically and emotionally exhausting for her. We discovered that this patient actually had an undiagnosed underactive thyroid. Once we treated that, the couple became pregnant. They even had to come back to the clinic to say, 'Dr Ryan, can you stop us from getting pregnant?'

That experience fascinated me and started what was to become a lifelong passion. It also showed me how much we need to teach both doctors and patients about hormonal health. That woman could have been saved from so much heartbreak had her thyroid issue been diagnosed earlier.

It's such a fascinating topic but it's something that has not been researched nearly enough. It affects so much of what happens in our bodies, particularly for women. All of the big life changes that happen in a woman's body – puberty, perimenopause and menopause – are a direct result of hormonal changes and yet so little is still known or discussed. In addition to the hormone cycle going on with their period, they also have their pituitary gland regulating every other hormone, so this whole hormonal vortex is interlinked on every single day of women's lives. This has never been fully appreciated.

I am passionate about education. It is the most empowering gift that we can give ourselves. I have spent the last few years travelling the length and breadth of the country speaking at conferences and talking about hormonal health on the radio, in newspapers and magazines and on television in the hope that we can raise awareness about these powerful medical messengers that control so much of our health.

When we understand our bodies and what they need for good hormonal health, especially for women, we can advocate for ourselves, at home, at work and in the doctor's office. For too long, we didn't have the information we needed to be in control of what was going on in our bodies. There was embarrassment and shame around the subject and women were often expected to live in pain.

I have been working to change that, to educate and empower women, and those days are thankfully behind us now. We can look forward to a future where open conversations about women's health and hormonal health are normal and we are able to understand our bodies more.

I am glad to have played a role in that conversation and I hope that by the end of this book you will understand how your hormones shape your health. I want you to feel confident in your ability to know your body and be able to identify any changes.

You are your own best advocate when it comes to your health, and you know yourself better than anyone else. Above all, I hope that you will put yourself first, give yourself time to rest, and prioritise your well-being.

It is time to learn how to say no with a smile and treat yourself the way you treat everyone else.

It is also time to turn your gaze on yourself first before you put it on others.

CHAPTER ONE
Why We Need this Book

Have you ever said any of these sentences to yourself?

- I'm exhausted, maybe I just need a tonic.
- I wonder if everyone has this much pain every month.
- Why am I so angry?
- Why don't I want to have sex with my partner?
- Do I have early dementia?
- Do I need hormone replacement therapy?
- Why can't I sleep?
- Why am I putting on weight?
- Am I diabetic?

If you have, you probably need to visit an endocrinologist like me. For men and women, but particularly for women, hormones play a huge role in our health and well-being.

For generations, women have been taught to say nothing about our health, to keep quiet and carry on. Periods were not discussed; menopause was just something that happened, and exhaustion was par for the course. None of that is good enough. How do you know what is normal and medically correct if you can't openly discuss it?

I am all for speaking openly, frankly and, some would say, loudly about hormonal health and how everything we do in our lives, from how much we sleep to what we eat and how we deal with stress, impacts our well-being.

How hormones affect physical and mental health

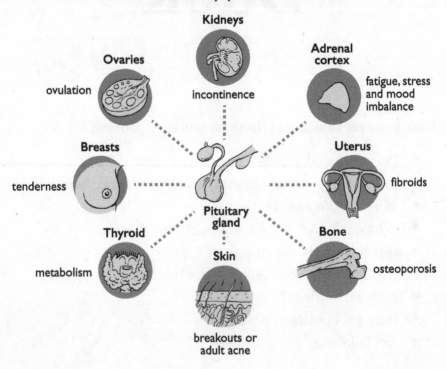

There have been great strides in women's health in Ireland in the last decade but much of that has come directly from women's own insistence that we must be listened to. On International Women's Day in 2022, the very first Women's Health Action Plan was launched. It included additional funding for the continued implementation of the National Maternity Strategy, a €9 million fund to enable women aged 17 to 25 to access free contraception, the first Maternity Bereavement Survey, legislation to strengthen the regulation of assisted human reproduction, additional breastfeeding support, expanded eating disorder services, four specialist menopause clinics and two specialist endometriosis services.

At the launch of the plan, Orla O'Connor, Director of the National Women's Council and member of the Women's Health Taskforce, said: 'The Women's Health Taskforce made the conscious decision to put women's voices at the heart of health policy and implementation, and this Plan seeks to deliver on what many women shared through the "Radical Listening" exercise – an ask for a person-centred and accessible health system, which works to meet women's needs as they arise. This Plan provides strong steps towards building that future for women in Ireland and our task is now to drive forward these actions that will be the critical levers for delivering meaningful change.'

We are our own strongest advocates, but to be in control we must be educated, have the facts, and openly discuss what goes on in our bodies so that we know what is normal.

A great example of that is our period. A menstrual cycle is something that half the population experiences and so the idea that periods are taboo or embarrassing is ridiculous. They are just part of millions of women's normal lives. Education and discussion around normal periods could alleviate so much suffering around endometriosis, polycystic ovary syndrome, fertility and much more.

I see things changing, but that change is still too slow. In 2022, Minister for Education Norma Foley put forward a proposal for an updated version of the Relationships and Sexuality Education (RSE) curriculum. This was the first change in 20 years. Think how much the world has changed in that time! Women and men should be taught about women's bodies from an early age and tampons, sanitary towels, mooncups and period pants should just be part of the conversation. There should be no more shame or embarrassment. Periods should be celebrated instead of being seen as a nuisance – they are necessary to create the egg that will fertilise with a sperm and create a miracle child.

When I began educating people about hormonal health, I started doing lectures all around the country with TV presenter Lorraine Keane. She is a warm host and a popular, well-known personality so I knew that she would get women into the room and that getting them there was half the job. Up until that point I had been educating GPs and medical students, but I felt that it wasn't enough.

I knew that public education was the key and I wanted to be able to speak to women about hormonal health and start a conversation about perimenopause and menopause so that they could go to their doctor and say, listen, this is what I think is going on, these are my symptoms and we need to sort this out together. Many of the subjects I was speaking about were taboo and women were embarrassed to speak about their sex lives, their periods or changes to their bodies. Women's issues, as they were often called, were deemed too private to speak about, which I think was just a way of silencing women.

All too often, if a woman was brave enough to broach the subject she was fobbed off and I was tired of hearing the same story. If they were brushed aside or not listened to, I wanted them to be able to confidently say no, I know that what is going on is not normal for me, it is probably related to my hormones and I want you to listen to me and help me. I wanted women to know what they were dealing with so that they could advocate for themselves.

We know that women's health concerns and pain are not treated the same way as those of men. In a study published in the official journal of the Society for Academic Emergency Medicine, it was found that women who attended the emergency department reporting acute pain were less likely to be given opioid painkillers than men with the same complaint. It might seem strange or shocking now that we needed actual roadshows about women's health but, up until very recently, nobody was speaking about it openly.

I could see from the women coming to speak to me in my clinics that far too many of them didn't know what their menstrual cycle should be like. They were coming into me absolutely exhausted and with severe anxiety and no one had ever asked them anything about their cycles.

Far too often, women come into my clinic with painful periods that last five or six days and have no idea that this is not the norm. They have been suffering unnecessarily for years because there is no discussion around the subject. I felt I needed to get out and speak to women about what a normal period is. It is shocking to me that even to this day some women do not realise that they don't need to suffer, that a normal period is supposed to be three or four days long with pain on the first day and slight cramps over the next few days. It is not normal to be doubled over in pain, get sick with period pain and have to lie on the floor because of it.

Women are passing huge clots and thinking that it's normal. How many of us know (or indeed are) women like that? Women who just put up with disruption to their lives and are never listened to?

I'm sure a lot of you have had someone tell you to hug a hot water bottle and get on with it. You could be crippled, unable to go to school or work, taking painkiller after painkiller and led to believe that it is normal, that everyone goes through it and it's just part of being a woman. That attitude to women's pain and health is not good enough.

I want young women to know that if their period is longer than three or four days it means that there's a hormonal problem that needs to be sorted out. If we're able to help young women, we are preventing fertility problems down the road. We're helping with the process of diagnosing endometriosis and we're also giving that poor adolescent girl a good quality of life. Imagine telling a child, because that is what they are, that a lifetime of pain is normal for women and something to get used to. How many times have I heard women say my life was great until I got my period and since then it has been hell? Unfortunately, most of those who were saying that to me were in their late 30s.

There is such power in young women taking control of their bodies and being able to investigate things that are going wrong years before the heartache of infertility or endometriosis. So many women have been told to put up with heavy, painful periods until they conceive and that having a child will sort it out. The inhumanity of telling a woman to live their life in pain until they can get pregnant is shocking. And there should be no presumption that every woman wants a family.

The more we know about our hormonal health the more we can step up and say no, I need tests, I need intervention. Being empowered with knowledge means that women can go to their doctors and demand the treatment they deserve.

But I also think that education must include boys and young men. If we want all aspects of women's health to be normalised, we need our young men to see it as normal, not embarrassing or dirty. We want young men to go into the shop and buy sanitary products without shame, we want them to understand what we go through so that they can be empathetic and helpful. We really must include men in conversations about periods, fertility and menopause.

Periods have been around since Adam and Eve. And it feels like women have not been listened to since then as well.

Endocrinology

Now, you might say, that's all well and good, but what is endocrinology? If you have never had diabetes or a problem with your thyroid, you may never have heard of an endocrinologist.

While endocrinology does deal with diabetes and thyroid disease, it also deals with all hormones. Traditionally, it had a narrow focus because not enough research had been done into all the other hormonal areas. But as we gain more and more knowledge about the role of hormones in overall health, endocrinology is starting to be valued as the important area that I've always known it to be.

Like so much else in the world, I believe it took women coming into medicine to focus attention on the role of hormones in general health. The problems were always there; they're just being discussed, researched and recognised at a much higher level now.

How do we know when something is off?

What we're going to do in this book is to help you understand and know your body. Once you have all the information you will be better able to recognise when things aren't running in the way that they should.

Women are often worried that they're going to be seen as a hypochondriac if they report everything they feel is wrong, but remember that everything is linked, so ignoring one thing might trigger another thing. You're much better off going to see your doctor, even if it's only for peace of mind.

For women, a lot starts with our menstrual cycle. If our periods are off, that's generally a sign that there's something up. If your periods get too heavy or become irregular, that could be a sign that you're overtired, or that the thyroid isn't functioning correctly, because everything is linked together.

If bowel motions change, which is something a lot of people ignore, that could also be a sign because hormones control the bowel muscle.

If you're not sleeping right, that could be a sign of hormonal imbalance.

If you have headaches, that could be a sign because, again, hormones control muscles so an imbalance of hormones at the nerve muscle junction will cause headaches.

Headaches, tiredness, change in bowel motions, not sleeping well and period changes are the first big indicators for women, and they are what I look for first. If you learn how to take the time to listen to your body, you'll start to see the subtle signs. Things generally run quite smoothly, so any change is something to note. If you need to, keep a diary of symptoms on your phone or in a notebook so that when you go to your doctor you have a record. I value a good consultation, as listening to what a patient says is very revealing to me. If you're able to give me detailed symptoms or changes, all the better.

Everybody laughs at the idea of man flu, but really, men have the right idea. They recognise that they're not feeling 100%, they say so and they take the time to rest. It's the most sensible thing in the world and we only laugh at it because it's such a foreign concept to us.

As women, we often try to power through until we're dead on our feet. But who is really right in that situation? We must change and start tuning into ourselves.

We are amazing nurturers, and we have amazing intuition which we've been given biologically, but we don't always listen to it. We need to trust our gut. If something feels off, it probably is, and if you're feeling tired, you must lean into that.

We are great at telling everyone else to rest and mind themselves, but we need to learn to take that advice for ourselves. Once again, we must start turning our gaze on ourselves.

Exhaustion

One of the biggest problems I see in my clinics is exhaustion. We are all tired sometimes, but exhaustion is a tiredness that impacts our lives. It's where you can't get up or do the jobs around the place you used to do, where you feel like crying with tiredness.

I see it in both men and women but as women, we're often programmed to do the most we possibly can. We're trying to balance home life, work life, relationships and children, minding elderly parents and being everything to everyone. We're hardwired to keep going until we collapse.

It's an intergenerational problem that we need to break. Even though we've moved so far forward, we still tend to repeat the patterns of our mothers and grandmothers. Many women continue to work at full throttle, without delegating and without rest, and that is bad for all of us. We need to stop those dysfunctional intergenerational patterns so that we can have a healthy hormonal balance; and healthier people means a healthier society.

There's a fantastic positive and negative feedback system that goes on in our pituitary gland, the master control gland. It's like an amazing computer and we could never replicate it, but if it's not recharged, it won't work. I will speak more about this later in the book.

How many of us understand what is happening inside our bodies when we're exhausted? Some reach for a tonic, some for a glass of wine at the end of the week, but not enough of us consider what we really need, which is a good rest.

If women overdo it, and they often do because they don't know how to ask for help, they end up burning out. They've utterly exhausted their hormones and on top of everything else they're having periods every month or they're going through perimenopause and menopause and that in itself means there's a hormone flux going on in that hormone control centre.

I am sure you know (or indeed are) that woman who will always just keep going when they're tired instead of sitting down and allowing the pituitary gland to recharge. Exhausted women come to my clinics and I'll ask them why they don't sit and take a break or have a rest. They always tell me, 'I'm trying, doctor, but I feel desperate when I stop.'

Well, of course they do, because once they stop, the whole train collapses, which is exactly what it needs to do. It's your body's way of saying that you have to stop, but women rarely listen to what their body is trying to tell them. They've seen their mothers battle through, or they are doing everything for their children and won't rest until it's done. They rarely take a break to think about the damage they're doing to themselves. They worry that someone will think they're lazy. You're not lazy if you're tired – your body is screaming at you to rest and you need to listen to it.

Modern technology is a wonderful thing and I see a lot of patients with smartwatches who can tell me that they're only sleeping for two hours and that they regularly have poor-quality sleep, and I'm not surprised. If you're only getting a quarter of the eight hours your body needs to operate then your pituitary gland and your adrenal glands are not going to be recharged. What I find fascinating is that all these people who come to me, who present me with this incredible technical data, do nothing about it. Having all that information right there on their wrist isn't making them rest!

When you're as tired as that, all your circadian rhythms are off, and that's why these patients feel as exhausted as they do. That's why they get aches and pains, headaches and brain fog. People very rarely see the link between tiredness and their brain, but if everything in your body is tired that includes your brain. Everything slows right down and that means that the synapses in your brain slow down too.

Women come to me in a panic, telling me they have early-onset dementia. They can't remember people's names, they are reaching for words and they're, quite naturally, devastated about it. I ask them some questions, talk to them about their lives and quickly discover that the real problem is that they are absolutely exhausted.

I see a lot of patients with chronic fatigue, which is a debilitating condition that is incredibly hard to live with. I primarily see it in women and for too long those women were given a raw deal because it was dismissed as being in their heads, but it's a very real condition.

Chronic fatigue is when the hormonal system is exhausted. The pituitary gland is tired, the adrenal glands are tired and, as a result, all your circadian rhythms are off. What's intricate and amazing about hormones is that they work in a circadian rhythm, so it's all closely timed.

Depression

I think that for too long women have been fobbed off and told that they're being over the top or that it's in their head or that they're depressed. I believe that depression is over-diagnosed in women; it's often used as a quick answer to a deeper problem.

I was very lucky to have had the late Professor Anthony Clare lecture me in psychiatry when I was a student and he used to talk about reactive depression and endogenous depression. He said that endogenous depression is true depression, a complete chemical depression where people are sitting in a chair, they have no insight, and they just can't get up. They're completely unable to do it, and life is very difficult for these patients.

However, reactive depression, sometimes called situational depression, is caused by a hormonal imbalance. It can be caused by a traumatic event, stress, or by running on empty. So many women suffer from this when they are exhausted, stressed, having heavy periods or are up all night with children. Their pituitary gland is tired and so everything is out of sync and suffering as a result.

For example, if you have very heavy periods that last five or six days, that will eventually wear out your hormonal system, and you're going to end up going to the doctor with severe fatigue because that affects your pituitary gland. The FSH and LH (follicle-stimulating hormone and luteinising hormone – we'll speak more about both of these a little further on) that control the whole cycle originate in that master pituitary gland. If your FSH and LH are off and you're getting over-long periods, that means your pituitary gland is going to be affected and that has a knock-on effect.

By the time I see a patient like that they need to be prescribed more than just rest. They might be at the stage where they can't sleep at all because they're so exhausted and the hormonal system is so far gone. As a result, there's too much adrenaline in the system because the adrenal glands are pumping adrenaline trying to get muscle receptors to pick it up. Of course, the receptors don't, and adrenaline goes into the bloodstream and then you get palpitations and sweating.

That's the stage where I get women coming to see me who are only in their 30s questioning whether they're in perimenopause because they can't sleep and they're experiencing severe sweating. They're nowhere near perimenopause; their entire system is just completely exhausted.

In those cases, I'll have a look at everything, and we'll see what needs to be fixed. In a lot of cases, the thyroid might be off because, remember, your master gland controls that as well. So I might have to fix those hormones with medication in addition to getting the patient to learn how to rest.

The one thing I ask women to do is to listen to their bodies, and this is where learning to prioritise yourself comes in. Remember that you're important too. Pull back, and instead of doing what every woman does, which is to keep going, you've got to take time out and rest. It's not a game.

Guilt

I have always found that guilt is a female phenomenon. I see it every day in my clinic. Did you ever wonder why women always feel guilty if they are away from their families when they are working? I never have met a male patient who feels guilty about being away from his wife or children, but it is endemic to us.

There are conversations all around the world right now about how women should balance their family and their career. Very few people are having that conversation with men, and I'd like that conversation not to be happening at all. When two people decide to start a family, two people are responsible for that family equally, and if one person decides to stay at home with the children, and I firmly believe that is one of the hardest jobs there is, they should get holidays, time off and help with all the other jobs around the house too. Partners must be equal.

We need to start this conversation in our primary schools. Our children watch everything we do and learn from it every day. It's so important for them to see a mum who looks after herself and puts herself first. Psychologists tell us that up to the age of seven boys and girls see themselves as equal. After that, the disparity becomes apparent to both and this affects their empowerment of self and their self-worth. If we want our children to see strong women, that starts at home. It will help your children, it will help you and, ultimately, it will help your health.

My own life

I often get asked if I'm good at taking my own advice. I know that from the outside I look very busy, I'm all over the country doing talks and events, I'm running my clinics and I have three children at home. But rest assured, I do take my own advice. I'm very good at going to bed early; I can't cope with lack of sleep, I really need my rest, so I go to bed early and I sleep really well. I have great energy and I'm very thankful for that. I cope very well with stress too so that helps a lot. I also get a great buzz out of the job so I'm lucky there as well.

I am very aware that I'm giving out a lot of advice to my patients, telling everyone to not do everything, to rest and to mind themselves, and so I do try to practise what I preach!

Because I've been telling patients about the need for rest for so long, listening to my own body is second nature to me now. I have been blessed with fantastic energy but I'm human like everyone else. I do overdo it on occasion, and I can feel a crash coming when I do.

The difference, I suppose, is that I listen to my body and when I crash, I go with it. It's important to hear what your body is telling you so there are weeks where I've pushed too hard and I need to spend the weekend minding myself. I make sure I eat well and get a lot of sleep.

I think when you're a very capable person and used to just getting on with things and powering through your list you expend a lot of energy without even realising it.

I know a lot of very capable women and they're all the same. It's part of that 'oh it's just easier if I do it myself' attitude. It may be quicker but you're not doing yourself any favours. Capable people probably use about three times more energy than anyone else so when they crash, they really crash!

I am also good at delegating. I had to get good at it because I became a widow nine years ago and I had to learn how not to do it all myself. I have a rota on the back of the door, and everyone in the house follows that.

Looking back on when my husband passed away, it was very tough. I think everyone who has gone through a bereavement wonders how they coped at the time. You're often in shock with a sudden passing, and you ask, 'What carried me through?' Everyone I've ever spoken to about it and every patient I've met since who has gone through a similar experience would say that they've asked themselves the same question.

For me, the children kept me going and work kept me going because everyone, even the patients, rallied around me. The love of the job and what I do helped a huge amount. I actually had to get my secretaries to stop patients asking me how I was doing when they came in because it would nearly set me back again. People are so kind, but I think I was just trying to plough through and keep everything together.

Really, though, you have no other option but to keep going. I had the children and they needed me to do that. My twin sons were eight and Una was only five and it was hard. I have a very supportive family as well and they were there to help me.

The one thing I always say to patients is to listen to your gut and to go with it. So I took my own advice. Whenever we were off work and school, I wanted to be gone; I just didn't want to be in the house.

Part of me did wonder what people were thinking of me. There she goes, she's run off abroad with the kids again. We always wonder what people think and I often tell people that it's nobody's business but yours what you do with your life. When you fully realise your self-worth, you will not care what anyone thinks and you will have arrived. More women need to do this.

When my children and I look back now we're delighted that we did it because it was a great way of bonding for all of us. We needed it because we were hurting so much and just being away as the four of us was what helped. I think learning to go with your gut is a big thing. You have to trust yourself. When you're grieving, you can feel completely exhausted and my way of coping was by getting away.

We always went to Lanzarote to a lovely hotel called the Rubicon Palace. Light helps our hormones and gives us energy and I got that when we went there. That hotel was a place I could get a bit of back-up, where I didn't have to be cooking meals or doing any of the usual home jobs. We needed the time out and we got it there. We also went to Orlando with a colleague of mine and got to go to Disney World. Building memories and having those times together really helped to get us through our trauma.

When I was home and working, delegating was what saved me. More women need to do this in their kitchens and make their children follow the rota of duties. It also empowers your children. You have to learn to do it and to speak up and ask for the help you need. I had great people around me and some wonderful babysitters to step in and mind the children.

We have the power to change our destiny

We each hold the power to change our future and take control of our health and wellness as much as we can. Our bodies and minds deserve care and attention and I think we know that more than ever after the global Covid-19 pandemic. Of course, we all get sick, that's life, but playing an active role in our well-being can minimise the risk and help to keep us healthy most of the time.

By understanding your hormonal system and empowering yourself to love yourself and know your self-worth you can banish your hormone woes for good and transform your life. If we're not good to ourselves, how can we expect other people to be good to us? If you don't think that you're worthy, other people may not think so either.

The key to self-care is in the word *self*. It is vital for your health, your mood, your work, your ability to focus, for lowering stress and for rest. All of that has a positive impact on your hormonal system.

We need to have the courage of our convictions and to learn to set boundaries. Boundaries are not there to keep people away, far from it; they're there to protect your energy and keep you feeling good.

Nourishing yourself starts with self-worth. If you know your value, you'll eat well, take time to exercise and get out into the fresh air, and you'll prioritise rest.

Spending time focusing on yourself each day is not a selfish pursuit. We cannot help others find success if we are not in top condition ourselves. We can transform our lives by loving ourselves, knowing our self-worth and thus allowing our hormonal system to take care of the rest.

A holistic approach

When patients come to see me, I recommend a holistic approach to identifying and understanding who you are as a person and then taking a seriously detailed look at the routines and lifestyle that landed you in your current predicament. Often people need to reset their lifestyles with self-care routines and rituals that help them rest, recover and reset so that their hormones are balanced. If you need medication too, that's fine, but it will work in tandem with your new routine and help you achieve full health faster.

We're all familiar with the old 'oh, she's just hormonal'. Well, yes, but we are all hormonal all the time and at some times more than others, as hormones keep our bodies functioning the way they are designed to. What we need to focus on is the ever-fluctuating balance of hormones in our own unique system.

Women feel pressured to carry the weight of the world on their shoulders, to strive to be all things to everyone in that world. Love, compassion and understanding – these are the qualities expected of us as we bend over backwards to care for and support our families, our friends, our co-workers and everyone who crosses our path. However, women often forget to care for themselves. Whose permission are we waiting for to be compassionate to ourselves?

If we push forward and constantly put others' needs above our own and we neglect to nurture our own needs, then we are the ones who suffer the consequences. Hormonal imbalance and mood swings ensue.

We ignore these symptoms in favour of pushing forward and maintaining our outward appearance of being in complete control. I am sure there are a lot of you ticking mental boxes while reading this – do not let yourself get to breaking point and do not let your foundations crumble until you become unrecognisable even to yourself.

You matter. Your emotional health matters. Your life matters. Your hormonal balance matters.

You deserve to treat yourself with the same love and compassion that you give to the world. Rebalancing, refocusing and reflecting on each day will help you stay in tune with your body, mind and soul.

That is why we need this book.

Your hormonal symptom checklist

Our hormones affect the way our body functions in almost every way. From your period and fertility to your weight, height and energy, everything is controlled by your hormones.

Here is a checklist of common hormonal imbalances and what to look out for. If you recognise any of these symptoms, it is worth speaking to your doctor or endocrinologist.

Polycystic ovary syndrome (PCOS)

- Irregular periods
- Hair growth on unusual areas such as the face, chest, abdomen and arms
- Adult acne
- Weight gain or difficulty in losing weight

Tests for PCOS include blood tests and an ultrasound to look for ovarian cysts.

Thyroid disorders

- Lack of energy, difficulty sleeping or exhaustion
- Racing heart or palpitations
- Changes to your period
- Sudden weight loss or weight gain
- Anxiety or low mood
- Changes to your vision
- A swelling or growth on your neck
- Unexplained hair loss

- Excess sweating or hot flushes
- Cold extremities (your hands or feet)

Blood tests are required to diagnose thyroid disorders.

Oestrogen imbalance

- Irregular periods
- Missing periods
- Very bad premenstrual syndrome (PMS)
- Breast tenderness
- Weight gain
- Exhaustion
- Pain during sex
- Migraines

Progesterone imbalance

- Irregular periods
- Missing periods
- Low libido
- Depression
- Difficulty in getting or staying pregnant

Prolactin imbalance

- Headaches
- Fertility issues
- Discharge from your nipples when not pregnant or breastfeeding

Chronic fatigue/pituitary fatigue/ ME (myalgic encephalomyelitis)

- Severe fatigue and lethargy
- Exhaustion
- Low blood pressure
- Inability to deal with stress
- Anxiety

CHAPTER TWO

The Endocrine System

We've all heard of hormones and at some point, many of us have been accused of being hormonal, which of course we all are, because at the most basic level hormones control everything.

As you learn more about hormones and their role in overall health and well-being you will begin to hear more about my speciality – endocrinology. The endocrine system is made up of all the hormones in your body and endocrinology is the study of what they do and how they impact our health.

Ernest Starling (1866–1927) was the first scientist to understand the significance of the endocrine system and to coin the word hormone. The system's existence had been described anatomically but no one really knew what hormones did. Thankfully, this is changing but there is a lot more to be researched to understand these amazing substances.

Hormones are little chemical messengers that are passed through the bloodstream and activate receptors. I like to think of them as the foot soldiers that get everything working. They're incredible, and you'll soon see why I chose to make them my life's work.

Hormones are vital for every organ in your body, and they control more than you could ever imagine. You already know that they are an important factor in your mood, your menstrual cycle and your fertility, but did you also know that they help to keep your brain agile, your bones strong and your immune system working? They're vital for digestion, blood flow, controlling your appetite and sleep. Do you see why I'm so fascinated by them?

Your hormones work by way of a positive and negative feedback system. If there's too much of one type of hormone, a message will be sent to the master control gland that there's enough there. It's a lovely rhythm, but for there to be balance in that system the hormone control centre needs to be well-rested – that's the key.

Adrenaline was the first hormone isolated in 1895. Since then, 100 hormones have been discovered. They are primarily produced in the hypothalamus (in the brain) and in the pituitary, thyroid, pancreas, adrenal and male or female reproductive glands.

There are also small quantities produced in the intestine. Some hormones are antagonists, acting to return conditions in the body to acceptable limits from opposite extremes. For example, insulin and glucagon keep our blood sugars in control. Hormones such as oestrogen and progesterone work together, and in pregnancy cause the lining of the uterus (the endometrium) to grow.

PMS

Hormonal changes are marked by extreme ups and downs. Your mood can escalate from being well to feeling anxious and apprehensive, as most women reading this book will know. For example, the monthly hormone fluctuations associated with premenstrual syndrome (PMS) give 80% of women who are menstruating nausea (sometimes severe), abdominal cramps and a depressive mood sometimes associated with irritability and anxiety.

Pregnancy and hormones

Hormone fluctuations are especially noticeable during pregnancy. How many of us are aware of pregnant women who have severe food cravings? That is all down to hormones. I recall when I was in the early stages of expecting twin boys I had to stop on the road on the way home to eat steak. I would never have the urge normally to eat steak and have that absolute need to stop to get it, but this time I just had to. I now know that I was low in iron as my twins were growing very fast inside me and I needed to replenish my iron levels.

The levels of oestrogen and progesterone are naturally high in pregnancy for several months as they ensure blood circulation in the pelvis, breasts and placenta to care for the growing baby. But then hormones drop rapidly after birth. This results in almost all new mothers suffering a hormonal imbalance between the second and tenth day after giving birth. This is often called the baby blues.

I had a severe episode of this when my twins were born. I worked too hard prior to their birth (which of course I tell all my patients not to do) and then one of my twin boys was critically ill with respiratory distress syndrome when he was born and on a life support machine, which added to my stress levels and hormonal imbalance. It was like I was in a dark hole. I was very low, I could not see a way out and was feeling very emotional. Within a few days, I felt better as a result of rest and seeing that my son was going to make it through. I got great support from the maternity nurses and staff in the Maternity Hospital in Limerick, to whom I will be forever indebted, and also from my family. That son who almost died is now 6 foot 5. What a turnaround!

We need to speak more about maternal hormones to support women around this time so they will not be wrongly labelled as depressed and also so their spouses and society can be there for them. Any of us can get a hormonal imbalance depending on what situation we are in and we need people to be there for us, but they also need to understand what we are going through.

This is why education about hormonal health and these amazing hormones that control everything in our bodies is so important. It is not just women who have hormones, of course – men have them too and we need to speak more openly and educate the public more so that both sexes can live a healthier life and know how to control their hormonal health.

The key to good hormonal health is balance. Too much or too little of a certain hormone can affect our health, as you will see. If some hormones are not performing, this will affect other hormones.

Of all the systems that work in our bodies, it is our hormones that work together the closest. They have an amazing regulatory system that is incredibly sensitive to many elements of our lifestyles.

The master control gland

The hormone control centre has another name – the pituitary gland. It's the master control gland and even though it is controlled by the hypothalamus in the brain, it's the pituitary gland that's in charge.

It's a small pea-sized gland at the base of your brain, behind your nose. It sends out signals to all the other organs. For example, it sends out the FSH (follicle-stimulating hormone) to the ovaries, causing the eggs to start maturating for ovulation. Your period actually starts in your brain – isn't that amazing?

If your pituitary gland isn't working as it should, it can affect lots of things in your body like your brain, mood, energy and vision.

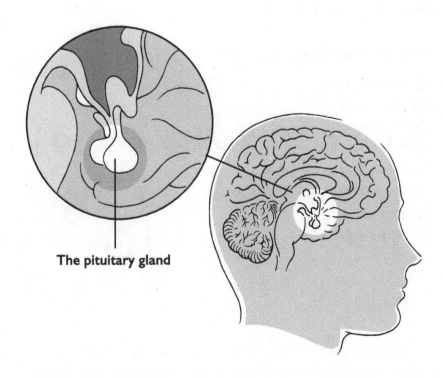

The pituitary gland

The hormones in your body are mainly produced in seven large glands: the hypothalamus and the pituitary, which we've already mentioned, the thyroid, which you're probably familiar with, the pancreas, the pineal gland, the adrenal glands and both the male and female reproductive glands (the testes and ovaries).

All sorts of messenger signals are sent out through the hormones produced in these glands. They control things like cortisol (the stress hormone), oxytocin (the cuddling hormone) and ghrelin (the hunger hormone).

Some of the hormones can have a dual purpose. Prolactin, for example, is secreted by the let-down of breastmilk, and when we're breastfeeding, we have high prolactin levels, but it can also be a stress hormone. If somebody's very stressed, prolactin levels go up. It can also be high in people who have epilepsy; if they have a seizure, prolactin is elevated.

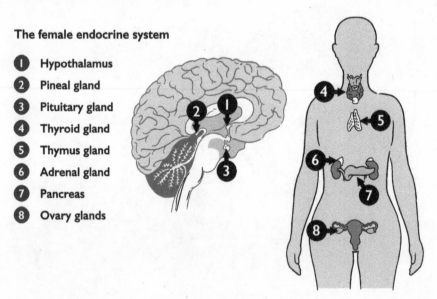

The female endocrine system

1 Hypothalamus
2 Pineal gland
3 Pituitary gland
4 Thyroid gland
5 Thymus gland
6 Adrenal gland
7 Pancreas
8 Ovary glands

The hormonal system is very complex and because of the positive and negative feedback system, a lot of it is intertwined.

One thing not working the way it should can have a huge knock-on effect in the body.

The main thing that causes this imbalance is exhaustion, which is one of the reasons I'm always asking my patients to rest when they're overtired. Your body needs that rest to recalibrate and find balance again.

I often liken an imbalanced hormonal system to an injured athlete. If they have a knee injury and they run on it they're going to delay recovery; the same is true if you have a tired pituitary gland.

It's a message that really needs to be heard more. Your pituitary gland needs rest to be recharged properly in order to work the way it should. There can be no underestimation of the amount of rest that is needed. You cannot expect your body to run on empty for prolonged periods of time and not react to that. Rest is always, always one of the first things that I prescribe and, believe me, I'm not above calling patients' family members to let them know that mam or dad or whoever it is needs to sit down with their feet up or get a good night's sleep!

Some key hormones and what they do

If we want to know our bodies and understand how they work, we need to be able to identify what is happening if something goes wrong. I firmly believe that a lot of good health lies in education. The more we know our bodies the more we can identify the small changes that might lead to bigger issues further down the road. The better informed we are the more in control we are. Here are some of the key hormones, what they do and what to look out for if there's a problem.

ADH

ADH is the anti-diuretic hormone (also known as vasopressin) and it regulates water balance and the sodium levels in your body. It's important for maintaining the volume of water in the space that surrounds our cells. Contrary to popular beliefs around hydration at the moment, it is possible to be overhydrated and that can result in an imbalance in your ADH levels. We all need 2 litres of water a day but the current craze for carrying around and refilling enormous water bottles may not actually be as good for you as you think.

Adrenaline

Most of us will be familiar with how the body reacts to a stressful situation. Your hands might start to sweat, your heart will race, and you'll be looking for a way out of the situation. This is the fight or flight response and that all comes from the hormone adrenaline. It's a crucial hormone but overexposure to it can be damaging to health in the long term.

During times of stress, adrenaline is quickly released into the blood which sends signals to organs to act in a certain way. The body's ability to feel pain is greatly reduced by the release of adrenaline, which is why you can run or fight even if you're injured. When the perceived danger has gone you can still feel the results of adrenaline for up to an hour.

It's an important part of how we survive in times of danger but sometimes your body will release adrenaline when it's under stress but not in real danger.

Cortisol

Cortisol is made in the adrenal glands and is known as the stress hormone, but it is also important for normal blood pressure, maintaining blood sugar levels and maintaining a normal metabolism.

On a normal day, your cortisol levels should decrease at the end of the day just as your melatonin levels are increasing so you can go to sleep. They stay low during the night and slowly start to rise in the morning to wake you up.

But primarily, cortisol is your body's main stress hormone. Your hypothalamus and pituitary gland can sense if there's the right level of cortisol in your blood. If it's too low, a message is sent to the adrenal glands to make more and adjust the levels released.

If your body is under stress, your cortisol receptors will use the hormone in different ways, where they think you need it most. They can shut down areas they deem unimportant at that moment, such as your digestive or reproductive system – that's why you might get a stomach ache when you're stressed.

When the stress has passed your heart rate and blood pressure should go back to normal and all should calm down, but what if you're under constant stress? That can lead to headaches, heart disease, weight gain, anxiety and trouble sleeping. Your immune system hates stress because cortisol decreases the number of immune cells in your body.

There have been studies done on all the things that can reduce our cortisol levels, such as massage, meditation and laughter. Try to devote at least 15 minutes of your day to stress-reducing activities. Make it a daily habit, something you could do when you wake up or in the evening as part of your night-time routine. Once you find something that works for you, you can start doing it whenever you feel a little stressed.

Dopamine

This is a neurotransmitter formed in the brain and the centre of the adrenal glands. Dopamine is the hormone responsible for keeping us motivated and driven for a long time. Drugs like cocaine extend the effects of dopamine.

Lack of dopamine can lead to Parkinson's disease, which causes symptoms such as a mask-like face, jerky muscle movements, tremors and a shuffling gait.

Endorphins

Endorphins are akin to the body's painkiller. They are formed in the spinal cord and the brain and also in white blood cells. They have an analgesic effect and dock onto opioid receptors (which mediate the body's response to most hormones, neurotransmitters and drugs). When you have an injury, endorphins protect the body from pain, but once that initial flood of endorphins wears off, the body recognises the pain related to the injury and collapses.

They are also released during stress. This is why people who work excessively get addicted to the short-term kick that stress gives them as stress releases endorphins.

FSH (follicle-stimulating hormone) and LH (luteinising hormone)

FSH promotes sperm production in men and stimulates the ovaries to produce oestrogen in women. LH stimulates ovulation in women and testosterone production in men. We'll hear a lot more about both of these later.

Ghrelin and leptin

These are the hunger hormones and are there to balance your natural appetite. You need rest in order for them to work properly, which is why you get really hungry when you're overtired. Ghrelin is formed in many places throughout the body, but it works directly on the brain. It induces the release of growth hormones (see below) and influences our dietary habits, moods and sleep. Its mode of action is complex, but basically, ghrelin production decreases when we eat, and the hormone oestradiol (see below) sends signals to the brain that we're not hungry anymore. When oestrogen levels are lower these messages don't work as efficiently, which is why your hunger levels might be different in perimenopause and menopause.

Leptin levels are regulated at night, which is why we're not hungry when we sleep. If you're not getting the right amount of sleep, your hunger levels won't be balanced, and again this can happen with sleep disturbances in perimenopause and menopause.

Leptin is formed by fatty tissue. It is passed into the blood and then reaches the satiety centre of the brain, making us feel full. It encourages fat cells to supply the body with energy, thus emptying or shrinking the fat cells.

Failure of the satiety centre to react to leptin is known as leptin resistance. This is one of the main reasons for obesity. Research has discovered that exercise can help in cases of leptin resistance.

Growth hormone

This helps to maintain healthy muscles, tissues, organs and bones and manage fat distribution. It is also the hormone that fuels childhood growth. It is produced in the pituitary gland.

Insulin

Insulin is one of the main hormones that an endocrinologist deals with. It is made by the pancreas and is sent into the bloodstream so that it gets to lots of different parts of the body. It has many effects, but its main job is to control how the body uses the carbohydrates found in foods. When carbohydrates are broken down in the body, they produce a type of sugar called glucose, which is the main source of energy used by our cells.

Insulin enables cells in the muscles, liver and fat to take up this glucose and use it as a source of energy so they can function properly. Without insulin, cells are unable to do this and start malfunctioning. The extra glucose that the cells don't use is converted to fat and stored so that it can be used for energy when glucose levels are low.

In healthy people, the release of insulin is tightly controlled in order to balance food intake and work with the needs of the body.

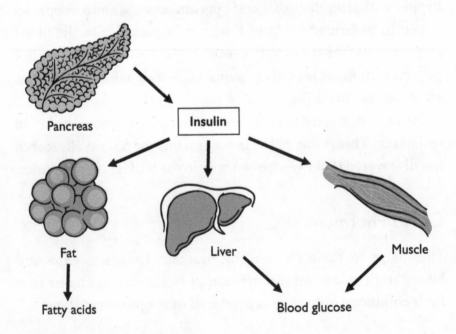

Diabetes

There are two types of diabetes: Type 1 and Type 2. People with the condition have problems with either making insulin, how insulin works in their bodies or both.

People with Type 1 diabetes produce little or no insulin. When you have too little insulin the body can't move glucose from the blood into the cells, which causes high blood glucose levels. People with Type 1 diabetes need to inject insulin to live.

Type 2 diabetes can be caused by two main factors. The person's cells may have difficulty producing enough insulin or the areas in the cells where the insulin acts become insensitive and stop responding.

Some people with Type 2 diabetes have very few symptoms initially and their condition is only found when they have blood tests for other reasons. Some people, however, experience symptoms very similar to Type 1 diabetes, such as thirst, frequent urination, dehydration, hunger, fatigue and weight loss.

Some people with Type 2 diabetes find that they can control their symptoms by improving their diet and lifestyle, but some will need medication and others may need to inject insulin. It is important to note that Type 1 diabetes is not caused by poor diet, weight or lifestyle. It is a chronic medical condition.

If you've ever been pregnant, you may have heard of gestational diabetes in pregnant women, which requires a glucose test in the hospital for diagnosis. The condition usually resolves itself after the baby is born.

Now, let's go back to stress. Hormones, like adrenaline, that are released into the bloodstream when your body is stressed stop the release of insulin, which leads to higher levels of glucose in the blood.

When your body is stressed the liver also produces more glucose so that you have extra energy. Whatever is not needed should get reabsorbed into the body, but that doesn't always happen. People who are more at risk of Type 2 diabetes and hyperglycaemia (when there is too much glucose in the blood) start to lose the ability to deal with insulin and eventually become insulin resistant. This resistance is also seen in conditions such as obesity and polycystic ovary syndrome. I'll talk more about the different types of diabetes in Chapter Seven.

Exercise and physical activity can have a strong impact on insulin levels in the body. Things like aerobic exercise, strength training and endurance exercise have been found to increase insulin sensitivity and reduce insulin levels. Even something as simple as regular walking can have a positive impact on these levels.

Melatonin

This hormone is produced by the pineal gland in the brain and its function is to regulate your sleep–wake cycle. It is produced in response to darkness and is affected by how much light you are exposed to before bedtime; exposure to too much light in the time before going to bed can block its production.

Melatonin is produced from serotonin. It is made in the pituitary gland, the intestine and the retina. During the night the immune system dedicates itself to cell reparation. The brain continues to learn as we sleep and our memory is trained.

Melatonin production begins to decrease from around the age of 30. This is one of the reasons why women can experience insomnia during menopause as it is connected to the lack of melatonin.

A good bedtime routine is really important to keep melatonin at its optimum level. Things like staying away from the blue light emitted from electronic devices before bedtime can help.

Oestrogen and progesterone

Oestrogen and progesterone are the ultimate female hormones. They cause breasts to grow in puberty and hips to become fuller; they control menstruation and make pregnancy possible. They also make sure we have strong hair and smooth skin. The long shiny hair that a lot of young girls have is a demonstration of this.

Oestrogen controls the female cycle, increases blood circulation in the uterus and improves bone density. It has a positive effect on blood lipids by increasing your good cholesterol (HDL) and lowering your bad cholesterol (LDL).

Oestrogen has nurturing qualities. Throughout history oestrogen in new mothers has ensured the survival of newborn babies. Oestrogen also ensures a cheerful disposition and emotional balance. However, our character is not only shaped by sex hormones but also by cortisol, which is produced by the adrenal glands and makes us more aggressive and stressed. Oestrogen affects our levels of happiness and our emotional equilibrium and progesterone affects our cortisol levels and calms our nervous system.

Oestrogen holds immense power in the sea of hormones. When our oestrogen levels are in balance, we feel calm, clear-headed and energetic. When they are off balance, we feel that our nerves are shredded. Oestrogen is produced primarily in the ovaries, in the fatty tissue, in a small amount in the testicles and in a region of the brain that is important for memory and learning. The hormone acts like a neuroprotective antioxidant, protecting nerve cells and their connections by intercepting aggressive and damaging molecules and proteins. Therefore, it protects our brains.

Oestrogen also stimulates blood flow, strengthens the immune system and stimulates the production of proteins leading to an increase of triglycerides (providing energy between meals) and cholesterol (helping the body make cell membranes) in the blood and water retention in the tissues.

Oestrogen receptors have antiproliferative and anti-inflammatory effects: they can stop cell growth and inhibit inflammation.

Oestrogens also protect against atherosclerosis, cardiovascular disease and Alzheimer's disease. From the age of 65, women are twice as likely to be diagnosed with Alzheimer's as men. We now know from research that this illness particularly affects the hippocampus, an area of the brain where oestrogen production drops dramatically during menopause.

High oestrogen levels are linked to a higher risk of thrombosis and some types of cancer and to being overweight. Excess oestrogen can also lead to liver damage.

Progesterone is the second most important female sex hormone as, on the one hand, it complements oestrogen and, on the other hand, it is its antagonist. Progesterone balances our oestrogen and without oestrogen, progesterone cannot fully take effect. Together they determine the menstrual cycle, make conception possible and allow an embryo to develop by protecting the mucous membrane of the uterus.

Progesterone is produced in the follicle cell from cholesterol. Progesterone acts not only on the uterus but on almost all body tissues in the brain as well as the peripheral nerves, essentially your arms and legs. It is important in energy production, the immune system, temperature and water regulation, and bone and fat metabolism.

It lowers the risk of various types of cancer and intensifies the effect of thyroid hormones. Together with oestrogen, progesterone protects against osteoporosis and encourages new bone growth.

Progesterone has a calming effect and helps us sleep better. It acts as an anti-inflammatory and a diuretic and flushes out fluids and tightens connective tissue. It increases libido, especially around ovulation. Progesterone is also crucial to the production of testosterone (see below) in men. Allopregnanolone, a precursor of progesterone which is formed in the brain and spinal cord, has a protective role in the central and peripheral nervous system.

Oestradiol

Both men and women produce oestradiol, and it is the most common form of oestrogen present in females during the fertile years. Too much oestradiol can be a bad thing and can result in acne, loss of libido, depression and osteoporosis. Very high levels of the hormone can increase the risk of uterine and breast cancer, while low levels can play a part in weight gain and cardiovascular disease.

Oestrone

Oestrone is the type of oestrogen that is present in the body after menopause and is a weaker form of the hormone.

Oxytocin

Since we produce oxytocin when we fall in love, this lovely hormone is known by many names: the love hormone, the cuddle hormone and the happy hormone. It helps labour to progress, causes breast milk to flow, affects behaviour and social interaction and the bonding between a mother and child.

Prolactin

This is the hormone that causes breast milk to be produced after childbirth. It also affects hormones that control the ovaries and testes, which can affect menstrual periods, sexual functions and fertility.

Serotonin

Serotonin is produced in cells in the gut, nerve cells in the brain and blood platelets. It is a critical hormone that affects our mood, body temperature, blood pressure and appetite. It is also a relaxant and encourages the intake of nutrients into the intestine.

The amino acid tryptophan is required for the production of serotonin. The body cannot produce tryptophan so we have to get it from our diet.

Chronic stress leads to malfunction in serotonin metabolism and can result in hypersensitivity, insomnia, lack of appetite and aggressive behaviour. For serotonin to be produced in appropriate quantities we need good sleep patterns and good stress reduction strategies.

Testosterone

In men, this hormone is produced in the testes and it is important for the development of the male reproductive tissues such as the testes and prostate. It also promotes secondary sexual characteristics such as increased muscle and bone mass and the growth of body hair. Its other important job is in controlling the libido. Women have small amounts of testosterone in their bodies, and the ovaries produce both testosterone and oestrogen. In women, it assists in the growth, maintenance and repair of female reproductive tissues and bone mass. If you have an imbalance of testosterone, it can have a negative impact on your health and sex drive.

Having too much testosterone isn't usually considered a common problem in men. Levels of the hormone can vary dramatically over the course of a day, and a lot of what we know about abnormally high levels of testosterone in men comes from athletes who use anabolic steroids, testosterone or other performance-enhancing substances.

In women, the most common cause of high levels of testosterone is polycystic ovary syndrome (PCOS). It's a common disease that affects between 6% and 10% of premenopausal women. A high level of testosterone is just one of the hormonal issues linked to PCOS. I'll explain the others, and treatment, in Chapter Four.

Testosterone is something of a hot topic at the moment as it forms part of the conversation around perimenopause and menopause. Testosterone deficiency in women may lead to low libido, reduced bone strength, poor concentration or depression. It's not currently licensed for use in women in Ireland and is sometimes prescribed 'off licence'. Its effectiveness in helping with sexual or cognitive function among menopausal and postmenopausal women is being researched widely – something I welcome.

TSH (thyroid-stimulating hormone)

This important hormone stimulates the thyroid gland, which regulates metabolism, energy and the nervous system. Thyroid hormones play the biggest role in steering the metabolism. They are formed in the thyroid gland, a butterfly-shaped organ in front of the windpipe at the top of the larynx. The hypothalamus and pituitary gland regulate this very important organ: the hypothalamus sends its messenger, thyroid-releasing hormone (TRH), to the pituitary gland, which sends thyroid-stimulating hormone (TSH) to the thyroid; once it arrives at the thyroid cells, it facilitates the release of the thyroid hormone.

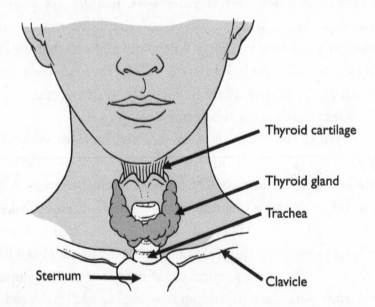

If you have ever felt run-down or very tired, it's likely that somebody will have asked you if you have had your thyroid checked and they'd be right to. It can impact lots of things like temperature, heart rate, mood, digestion, vision, sleep and appetite, and every aspect of your metabolism is regulated by thyroid hormones.

The thyroid gland produces two main hormones – thyroxine (T4) and triiodothyronine (T3). These two play a part in every cell in your body. They help to influence your heart rate and to regulate protein production, they influence how your body uses fats and carbohydrates and they help to control your body temperature. The thyroid hormones all contain iodine, which is why one of the thyroid's main tasks is the storage of iodine from our food. Ten per cent of T3 is directly produced as an active hormone in the thyroid. If required, it is converted from the inactive T4, which makes up 90% of thyroid hormone. This process of activation doesn't take place in the thyroid itself but in the intestine and liver.

If enough T3 and T4 are circulating in the blood, production of TSH from the pituitary gland is stopped. T3 is considered to be the biologically active thyroid hormone. It increases energy consumption and promotes the formation of the mitochondria, which are the power plants in our cells and increase muscle mass. It also supports the formation of other thyroid hormones including the happiness hormone serotonin as well as oestrogen, testosterone and progesterone. So as you can see, all hormones are interconnected.

If the thyroid level in the blood is in the optimal range, you will have lots of energy and feel strong, and your body will respond to behavioural changes such as increased exercise or a healthier diet. When your thyroid is working at its optimum you can regulate your temperature to suit all types of weather, your bowels work without grumbling, there are no problems with your libido, you have as much energy as you need and you are enjoying life.

If your thyroid is out of sync, however, you will experience insomnia, severe fatigue, digestion issues, lethargy and depressed moods. If your thyroid is not optimal, it makes conception very difficult, as I have seen on countless occasions.

Every thyroid hormone consists of the amino acid tyrosine and one or more iodine molecules. The various thyroid hormones are numbered consecutively according to the number of iodine molecules they have. Thus T3 has three iodine molecules and T4 has four. For T4 to become the active T3, an iodine molecule must be taken away. This requires an enzyme based on zinc and selenium. Around 60% of T3 is converted from T4 in the liver and around 20% in the intestine and the rest in the thyroid. This is another reason why we need to be good to our gut microbiome, as you will read about in Chapter Seven.

Women in the phase of hormonal change are particularly susceptible to thyroid disease. Therefore we need to nourish ourselves properly. Vitamin and nutrient deficiency, as well as alcohol, can prevent the conversion of T4 to T3. Other inhibiting factors are fasting, stress, medication, liver and kidney disease, progesterone deficiency during perimenopause, menopause and ageing. Alongside T4 and T3 there is also a lot of research into the thyroid hormones T2 and T1. A study in 2015 showed that T2 influences metabolism and body heat balance. Additional research is required in this area.

Thyroid disease is very common in women and that's because autoimmune disease is more common in women. An autoimmune disease is where the body attacks itself. Oestrogen can increase inflammation in the body while testosterone reduces it. Women also have a more reactive immune system which makes them less susceptible to general viruses but means that they are more likely to develop an autoimmune condition because of hyperimmune responses.

I believe that women are more likely to develop autoimmune disease due to a variety of factors including hormonal balance relating to heavy or irregular periods, perimenopause and menopause. When you add overwork and burnout to this mix the immune system is not as robust as it should be and you're at risk of autoimmune disease. I am convinced this is why we see more autoimmune disease in women compared to men. Interestingly, when I do see a man with thyroid disease it is almost always a result of burnout.

There are two main types of thyroid disease – hyperthyroidism (an overactive thyroid) and hypothyroidism (an underactive thyroid).

Hyperthyroidism

Hyperthyroidism is a condition where your thyroid makes and releases high levels of thyroid hormone. If you have an overactive thyroid, you may experience symptoms such as heat intolerance, poor sleep, anxiety, tremors, restlessness, weight loss despite no change in lifestyle, palpitations, diarrhoea, tiredness or changes in your menstrual cycle. If the condition is left untreated, it can lead to things like heart disease, heart failure, eye disease and, in severe cases, blindness.

An autoimmune disease called Graves' disease is sometimes the cause of hyperthyroidism. It is a condition that often runs in families where the immune system mistakenly recognises the thyroid gland as a threat and attacks it resulting in the oversecretion of thyroid hormone.

Graves' disease is named for Robert Graves, who discovered the overactive thyroid over 150 years ago. (He was appointed Physician to the Meath Hospital in 1822, which is where I trained and found my love for hormonal health!)

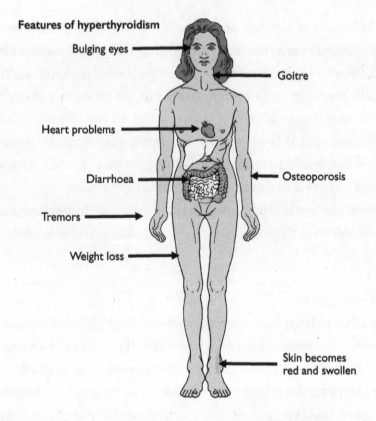

Features of hyperthyroidism

Bulging eyes

Goitre

Heart problems

Diarrhoea

Osteoporosis

Tremors

Weight loss

Skin becomes
red and swollen

Hyperthyroidism can result in several complications:

- Heart problems including palpitations, heart failure and
an irregular heart rhythm disorder called atrial fibrillation
that can increase your risk of stroke if it's not diagnosed in
time. If there's an irregular heart rate, you're more likely to
get a clot so it's very important to go to your doctor if you
notice this. Atrial fibrillation is the most common cause of
a stroke.
- Osteoporosis can also be a complication because untreated
hyperthyroidism can interfere with your body's ability to
incorporate calcium into your bones on which they depend
for strength.

- Some people with Graves' disease develop Graves' ophthalmopathy, which can cause eye problems including bulging, red or swollen eyes, double vision and sensitivity to light. If it is left untreated it can result in loss of vision.
- Graves' dermopathy is another condition of Graves' disease where the skin becomes red and swollen, most often on the shins and feet.
- A thyrotoxic crisis is where your symptoms suddenly intensify and lead to a high fever, a rapid pulse and sometimes even delirium. If this happens, you need to seek immediate medical assistance.

Hypothyroidism

Hypothyroidism leads to an increase in hormone production. Ninety per cent of hypothyroidism is caused by autoimmune disease which leads to chronic inflammation through the thyroid cells that are destroyed.

Hypothyroidism is sometimes caused by Hashimoto's disease, another autoimmune disease. Some people believe that they can cure Hashimoto's with diet alone, but that is not true and all patients need medication.

An underactive thyroid may present itself with symptoms such as:

- Tiredness
- Slow heart rate
- Oedema (excess watery fluid collecting in the body tissue leading to swelling)
- Low libido
- Sensitivity to cold
- Weight gain

It's Probably Your Hormones

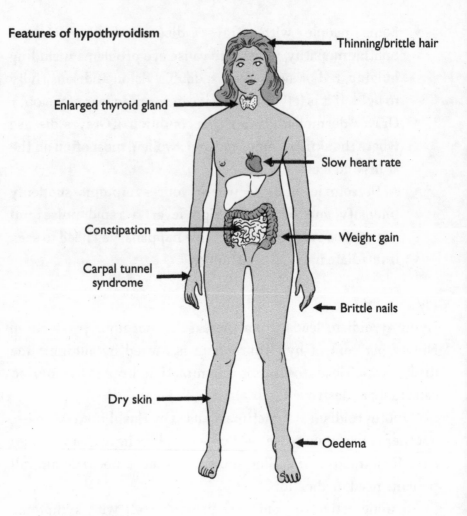

Features of hypothyroidism

Thinning/brittle hair

Enlarged thyroid gland

Slow heart rate

Constipation

Weight gain

Carpal tunnel syndrome

Brittle nails

Dry skin

Oedema

- Constipation
- Low mood
- Depression
- Forgetfulness
- Dry skin
- Thinning or brittle hair and nails
- Heavy periods
- Enlarged thyroid gland (also called goitre)
- Carpal tunnel syndrome

HASHIMOTO'S DISEASE

This is the most common form of hypothyroid disease and the second most common endocrine condition affecting women of reproductive age. It is also very common during perimenopause and menopause. It is assumed that one in ten women will get Hashimoto's disease during her lifetime. There is increased risk at times of hormonal change such as puberty, pregnancy and perimenopause.

Hashimoto's is caused by various chemicals and toxins, acute and chronic infections, flu and severe stress. Other triggers include food intolerances like lactose and gluten, leaky gut syndrome, a deficiency of magnesium, vitamin D and iron or a damaged microbiome caused by repeated antibiotic therapy.

At the beginning of the autoimmune process thyroid cells carrying hormones can be destroyed. Typically hyperfunction symptoms will become evident and then when the destroyed cells are empty the process swings into hypofunction.

With Hashimoto's in particular you get additional symptoms of hypofunction:

- Frequent throat clearing and coughing
- Hoarse voice
- Brittle nails and hair
- Neuropathic symptoms such as tingling and a burning sensation of the skin
- Irritability
- Digestive disorders
- Muscle pain and general weakness
- The feeling of a lump in the throat or pressure in the neck
- Carpal tunnel syndrome

Because of the many faces of Hashimoto's disease, it is often recognised too late. You need to check thyroid antibodies as well as TSH, T3 and T4. You also need a thyroid ultrasound. Thyroid antibodies are raised in 90% of patients with Hashimoto's.

Most Hashimoto's disease patients are treated with Eltroxin T4, while some need T3. I have seen patients with very low T3, which I call conversion disorder. When I saw a patient with this and gave her T3 and made dietary and lifestyle changes, she felt like a new woman in just a few weeks.

Another issue is reverse T3, which opposes T3 by attaching itself to the same receptor and blocking the effect of T3. If your reverse T3 levels are too high while T3 is normal, you will feel tired and lethargic. You can lower reverse T3 by abstaining from alcohol and nicotine, reducing stress and taking a combination of T4 and T3.

When do I take my Eltroxin?
Eltroxin interacts with certain foods and drugs and therefore the absorption can be reduced so that you do not get the desired effect. Therefore, you must take your thyroid medication at least half an hour before breakfast and any other treatments. I usually tell my patients to put them by the bedside and to take them first thing and by the time they have washed and dressed, they can take their thyroid medication.

Foods that are enriched with calcium like milk and dairy, orange juice, coffee, iron supplements, cholesterol-reducing drugs and proton pump inhibitors that we use for ulcers and gastritis can all interfere with thyroid medication.

Hashimoto's and gluten intolerance

It has been observed that the majority of Hashimoto's patients do not tolerate gluten well and suffer from gluten sensitivity or intolerance. It has also been shown that the antibodies that work against gluten can damage thyroid tissue, which is similar in structure.

Foods containing gluten, like wheat, barley and rye, produce an immune reaction in the small intestine that can be accompanied by an inflammation of the mucous membranes.

Consider the following if you have Hashimoto's disease:

- Probiotics for intestinal health
- Check for iron deficiency, as a good iron supply is essential for the production of thyroid hormones and the effectiveness of enzymes.
- Rule out iodine deficiency.
- Check your vitamin D levels are adequate.
- 200 µg of selenium – this lowers the amount of thyroid peroxidase antibodies.
- 25 mg of zinc – zinc is indispensable for thyroid function because it is involved in the activation of T3. Brittle fingernails, hair loss and reduced fertility are related to zinc deficiency.
- Vitamin B complex
- Avoid stress as high cortisol blocks the progesterone receptors.

When to get checked for hypothyroidism

You may not know you have an underactive thyroid at first. I often see patients present to me at the clinic with a range of other problems that they're trying to get sorted out. But people tend to have very usual symptoms and I know almost as soon as I start speaking to someone if we're looking at a thyroid issue.

If somebody came to me very tired, exhausted, with dry skin, dry hair and putting on loads of weight, I'd be very suspicious of an underactive thyroid.

Whereas if they came in and said they'd lost weight and had palpitations and sweating, I'd be fairly sure that we were looking for an overactive thyroid.

If you have any of the symptoms associated with an underactive thyroid, I would always recommend getting it checked. If left untreated, hypothyroidism can lead to a number of health problems that can cause a lot of difficulties.

Conditions associated with hypothyroidism include:

- **Goitre.** This is where your thyroid gland becomes enlarged due to constant stimulation. While it's generally not painful, it can affect your appearance and sometimes leads to difficulty swallowing or breathing.
- **Heart disease.** Because an underactive thyroid can mean that you have higher levels of LDL cholesterol (that's the bad one) hypothyroidism can lead to heart problems and is associated with an increased risk of heart disease and heart failure.
- **Depression** can occur early on in hypothyroidism and can become more severe over time.

- **Nerve damage.** If left untreated for a long time, hypothyroidism can cause damage to your peripheral nerves – the nerves in your arms and legs. This peripheral nerve damage may cause pain, numbness or tingling in the affected areas.
- **Fertility.** One thing I see in the clinic is fertility problems that are linked to an underactive thyroid. Low levels of the thyroid hormone can interfere with ovulation, which in turn affects fertility. Some of the autoimmune conditions that cause hypothyroidism can also have a detrimental effect on fertility. Your thyroid levels may not be the first thing you check if you're having difficulty in conceiving, but they should be.
- **Myxoedema.** This is a life-threatening condition associated with long-term, undiagnosed hypothyroidism. Symptoms of this rare condition include intense cold intolerance and drowsiness followed by extreme lethargy and unconsciousness. It can be triggered by infection, stress on your body or sedatives. If you have any signs of myxoedema you need immediate medical attention.

Treatment for thyroid disease

In the case of an underactive thyroid, treatment can be quite straightforward and the hormone is simply replaced through medication. An overactive thyroid can be a little more difficult to treat and can need extra treatment in a hospital.

CASE HISTORY: FIONA

Fiona was 38 when she came to see me. I see a lot of women who have been struggling to get pregnant for years and by the time Fiona made an appointment she had gone through five cycles of IVF. My heart went out to her. We all know how emotionally and physically difficult, and financially expensive, IVF is and to go through that five times without getting pregnant is dreadful. I really wanted to help.

We did all the tests and all her blood work and it showed she had hypothyroidism. Her FSH and LH levels told me that she wasn't anywhere near menopause, even though she was concerned that she might have early menopause because of her symptoms, which included severe fatigue and sweating. Her exam was normal apart from severe muscle pain in her arms and trapezius muscles, and she had restless legs. When nerve cells become damaged, the level of dopamine in the brain is reduced which causes muscle spasms and because dopamine levels fall at the end of the day the symptoms of restless legs syndrome are often worse at night. (Restless legs syndrome is a condition of the nervous system that creates a strong urge to move your legs when at rest.) Finally, she had a laparoscopy that showed that her fallopian tubes were fine.

It was time then to sit down and talk to her. When I probed, she admitted that she was very tired but she kept going because if she stopped and rested, she thought she might never get up again. She slept very poorly, she had aches and pains in her muscles and sweating and palpitations at night.

Once she told me that, I knew what we were dealing with. As an endocrinologist, I deal a lot with peripheral neuropathy in diabetes where the peripheral nerve function to the lower legs is affected and patients have burning feet and restless legs due to high blood sugars. People who have severe chronic fatigue/pituitary fatigue often present with the same symptoms.

I discovered that even though she was having periods, she was not ovulating. In other words, she had anovulatory cycles. There are times, such as if you have experienced loss or prolonged stress, when the body protects itself and does not ovulate as it knows that a period would be too much for the body to endure. When you are exhausted the body does the same thing and protects itself by not ovulating. We also see this in young girls who become underweight due to strict dieting.

I treated Fiona first for the underactive thyroid and her nerve pain – with a combination of medication and lifestyle changes – and then focused on explaining the importance of rest and recuperation. She did really well and went on to become pregnant.

CASE HISTORY: ANTHONY

I had been seeing Anthony, who was in his 40s, for a little while. He was under my care because he had Hashimoto's disease and his thyroid was underactive. He was also gluten intolerant, like many patients with Hashimoto's.

He was taking Eltroxin, a medication commonly used to treat Hashimoto's, and had done very well for several weeks, but was back to see me because his symptoms were returning. He was tired again and he had restless legs at night and wasn't sleeping well. I see this quite a lot. Patients start taking their medication, they change their lifestyle and they do really well, but then because they're feeling great, old habits start slipping back in.

I spoke to Anthony again about his lifestyle and cutting out the excesses. Our bodies are great at self-repairing when we allow them to, but if we overdo it we can expect the consequences. Anthony had gone back to his old way of doing things because he had done so well for the first few weeks on Eltroxin and thought he was cured.

Thankfully, that small relapse was the reminder he needed, and he took my advice about long-term lifestyle changes and pacing himself.

I'm glad to say that he did very well.

Pituitary fatigue/chronic fatigue

You might be familiar with terms such as chronic fatigue, post-viral syndrome, or myalgic encephalomyelitis (ME). They are all conditions where a patient presents with persistent fatigue that is not made better by rest and that has a profound impact on their work lives, social lives, friendships and lifestyle in general. They can also have other symptoms such as joint and muscle pain, sore throat, headaches and poor sleep.

It's an extreme tiredness that you wouldn't understand until it has happened to you, and it can be caused by viruses like Lyme disease or glandular fever or even Covid-19. In fact, a lot of the long Covid that we are seeing is similar to the symptoms of post-viral syndrome or chronic fatigue. In the 1980s scientists introduced post-viral syndrome as a description for patients who could trace their current illnesses back to a viral infection. It is basically a prolonged period of being unwell after having an acute virus and it's a good descriptor for what we're seeing now in patients after Covid infections.

But even though the textbooks call it ME or chronic fatigue, I prefer to use the term pituitary fatigue because I feel it provides a better explanation. I have had very sick patients come to me with profound fatigue, but once their hormonal imbalance is sorted, they do very well. Calling it chronic fatigue doesn't do the patient justice because they are severely exhausted, have severe muscle pain and disabling fatigue, and are frustrated by this fatigue. I have found that people are sometimes dismissive of such patients and this is wrong. It is a genuine illness that can be very debilitating for those experiencing it.

Patients are often passed off as being depressed but that is not the case. These are highly motivated people who often have to give up their careers because of the exhaustion. In my many years of dealing with this illness, I've seen that patients who suffer from this very disabling disease are exasperated at being so fatigued and very anxious to get back to normal. If indeed you did have endogenous depression, you would not be frustrated at being tired as you would not have that insight.

Pituitary fatigue is much more common in women than in men, though men do get it too. Aside from viral infections, there are some common reasons why I see pituitary fatigue more in women.

Having prolonged, heavy periods can be a factor. I often meet women who have very heavy, painful periods that can last seven days and have been suffering through that for 10 years or more. They might be working very hard at their career and then they have their first baby, are up all night with no sleep and a hormonal imbalance ensues.

I saw one such patient who had a history of seven-day periods which were very heavy and painful since puberty at 12. She then developed glandular fever at 18. She was a high achiever who went on to become a solicitor and was crippled with fatigue but kept going. She developed hypothyroidism and struggled to have a baby. During all this time she was pushing herself. When I met her at 37, I told her to go with the tiredness and pace herself. She had severe muscle pain and restless legs syndrome. She slept for the first time in years, allowing her pituitary gland and hormonal system to get back into their circadian rhythm. Eventually, I helped her to get pregnant and with the aid of a very supportive husband she managed to pull through. She did well during pregnancy but was exhausted after having the baby, as we so often see. Her husband took charge of the night feeds. She took extra time off and with the correct medical care and support and understanding from her family she eventually went back to work.

Another situation could be a woman who has taken a lot of hormonal treatment as a result of many sessions of IVF, leading them to be completely exhausted by the mental and physical exertion that takes. I have also seen it in women with very heavy periods. The minute they hit perimenopause the additional hormonal imbalance causes severe fatigue.

As a result of any of the above scenarios, the pituitary gland gets tired and the person ends up suffering from hormonal imbalance with severe peripheral nerve pain, sweating and palpitations. When the pituitary gland is tired, circadian rhythm and the rhythm of hormones are affected and you get excess adrenaline and low cortisol. As a result, these patients often present with sweating, palpitations and anxiety in addition to profound fatigue.

These women often ask me if they are in early menopause because they have only heard of their symptoms associated with that – nobody has mentioned pituitary fatigue to them. They don't realise that they are utterly exhausted. I have also seen this condition post-vaccination in some patients. This is because in some patients the inflammation caused by the vaccine causes a chronic inflammation; there may be underlying immune dysfunction in these patients that causes this. I have also seen this fatigue after severe infections such as meningitis, adenovirus infection and glandular fever (also called Epstein–Barr virus or EBV).

Symptoms of chronic fatigue/pituitary fatigue include:

- Severe lethargy
- Interrupted sleep
- Muscle pain
- Restless legs
- Irritable bowel syndrome (IBS)
- Headaches
- Brain fog

You may be surprised to see irritable bowel syndrome (IBS) in the list above. We know that the bowel is on average 8m long, wrapped up on itself. It is operated by hormones which control all muscles and works like a conveyor belt. However, when there is a hormonal imbalance this is affected and there is bloating, passing wind and belching. For too long we put IBS down to stress and dismissed patients, especially female patients, and told them that it was in their heads. But this is not the case. Instead, it is important to explain to such patients that the problem is caused by hormonal imbalance, immune dysfunction and chronic inflammation and not to dismiss them.

Long Covid syndrome

Most people who get Covid-19 recover within a few weeks. However, some will develop severe fatigue. This involves ongoing symptoms that people experience more than four weeks after getting Covid.

Symptoms of long Covid syndrome:

- Fatigue
- Fever
- Exhaustion after minimal exercise
- Shortness of breath
- Brain fog
- Insomnia
- Muscle pain
- Loss of smell and taste
- Anxiety
- Palpitations
- IBS
- Rash
- Changes in the menstrual cycle

A lot of these symptoms are similar to those caused by chronic fatigue which we would have seen with some patients after getting EBV or any serious infection that caused major inflammation or hormonal imbalance. I have also seen it in patients with endometriosis and a history of very heavy periods. Although EBV is a herpes virus, not a coronavirus, it has been speculated that another coronavirus, severe acute respiratory syndrome (SARS), might reactivate latent EBV and trigger the fatigue. In the SARS epidemic of 2002–4, 40% of sufferers experienced chronic fatigue.

In deciding how to act on long Covid, researchers and policymakers need to take heed of what happened in the case of ME. This condition shares the symptoms of long Covid and these patients have struggled for many years to be recognised as having a serious and debilitating medical condition that needs specialised treatment and research.

Hopefully, now there will be more research, and the recognition that long Covid has a very similar pattern to chronic fatigue/ME means that these patients will now be listened to and get the services they are entitled to. For example, a lot of these patients have to struggle to get income protection, as some insurance companies do not recognise ME. Perhaps now with the onset of long Covid insurance companies will have to do this, and the sooner the better as this *is* a real illness.

Pacing is key

One of the most important things I speak about to patients with chronic fatigue/pituitary fatigue is pacing. They have to learn to listen to their bodies and slow down. Yes, I treat the underlying hormonal issue, whether that's a problem with their thyroid or heavy periods, but fundamentally the objective is to get them to accept that they need to slow down. They need to walk, not run.

I come back to my injured athlete comparison here. If an injured player runs on an injured knee, they aggravate the problem. We allow athletes to take time to recuperate and we must treat ourselves in the same way. If you're run ragged, you cannot heal. If you expect your body to recharge while still running on empty, you're very much mistaken. It cannot happen. We all need a lesson in putting ourselves and our health and well-being first.

CASE HISTORY: GRÁINNE

Gráinne also came to see me when she had trouble getting pregnant. She was a busy woman in her late 30s with a career with a lot of responsibility and two children.

The first thing I did was ask her to recount her day to me.

She was getting up at 6 a.m. to do a workout and then working until 7 p.m. She would then come home, make dinner for her family, organise bedtime and then come downstairs to do more emails. When she went to bed she struggled to sleep because of restless legs. She described her energy level as 1 out of 10, 10 out of 10 being normal.

As soon as she mentioned restless legs, a lightbulb went on for me. That is very often a result of peripheral nerve root irritation when there is severe fatigue.

I explained to her the importance of getting more rest, giving up the workout for now, pacing herself and doing a regular day's work without all the extras in the evening. She was on the verge of burnout. She was given medication for the restless legs and I explained the importance of diet and healthy eating. We crave carbohydrates when we are tired, and she needed to cut out the extra sugar in her diet.

Three months later we checked Gráinne's progesterone levels and found that they rose at day 21, indicating that she had ovulated.

Once she became pregnant we spoke about her energy and managing her tiredness. Because she already had two children at home I was concerned about her trying to do it all. I am an advocate and supporter of breastfeeding, but in this instance, Gráinne opted not to breastfeed because if she became overtired again, she would be more likely to relapse. Breastfeeding is marvellous but we need to give new mothers plenty of support as they need plenty of rest around this time.

Pituitary fatigue is really like any other physical illness. If you have pneumonia you have to be careful of a potential relapse, and it is the same with pituitary fatigue. Breastfeeding is on demand and means interrupted sleep. This is fine if you're fit and healthy, but if you have already struggled and are at risk of relapse you need to be very careful. Remember, labour is a very long process that demands a great deal of energy, and at the end, you are immediately given a tiny baby to look after without any sleep, so your energy levels are already depleted.

CASE HISTORY: LAURA

Laura came to see me with severe fatigue that was disabling. An accountant in her 40s, she had two children aged 10 and 11 and had been completely exhausted since her second child was born. That child had had severe colic for a year and a half after he was born, and she got very little sleep during that entire time. She was also self-employed and trying to run a very busy business with her husband. She complained of severe muscle pain, brain fog, profound lethargy and insomnia and it was no wonder she was close to collapse.

Laura was very upset that her GP had suggested that she was depressed. She knew that wasn't it but she was frustrated with being so exhausted all of the time and needed help.

I asked her to list what she did on an average day and it included everything from making lunches for her children to doing all the household chores along with her busy job. She never once delegated at home or asked for any help from her children or her husband.

It is unsustainable to keep going like this but it took me pointing it out for her to see what was the root of her exhaustion. Sometimes you're just so preoccupied trying to get everything done that you can't see the problem.

Laura went on some medication to sort out her underlying hormonal imbalance. I spoke to her husband and children about helping out at home, giving her time to herself, drawing up a rota for the children and implementing it. The combination of the medication and the changes to her daily routine worked really well.

CHAPTER THREE
Menstruation

This is the chapter for you if you have ever pondered any of the following questions:

- Is my period normal?
- Does everyone get mood swings?
- How much bleeding is too much bleeding?
- Does everyone get cramps like me?
- Why do I crave sugar during my period?
- Do men know what's going on with periods?

I am adamant, passionate and very, very vocal about the fact that everyone should know what a normal period is. Girls are reaching puberty much younger than ever before and I want to save them from discomfort, pain and embarrassment by making periods a normal topic of conversation.

We are so far past the point in our society where dads should be embarrassed about going to buy tampons or making a joke about girls being moody because it's their time of the month. You can be sure that if periods were happening to young men we would *all* know about it.

So, what happens? The two hormones involved in menstruation are FSH (follicle-stimulating hormone) and LH (luteinising hormone). They are the two that control ovulation, and you know that when ovulation occurs on day 14 of the cycle the egg is waiting to be fertilised. If that doesn't happen it is released and you get a period on day 28. A normal period should last three to four days and if it is any longer than that there is a problem either with the secretion or with the hypothalamus. There is a hormone called GnRH (gonadotropin-releasing hormone) that is released by the hypothalamus that controls FSH and LH, and if that's out of sync it's going to cause problems with fertility down the road. So you can see why it's important to know early on if there's an issue.

One of the big problems that I see all the time is women with seven-day periods losing a lot of blood. We call it menorrhagia. If you have a period lasting more than five days and you find that you need to change your tampon, pad or cup every two hours or if you see very large clots, you may be experiencing menorrhagia. There can also be very painful cramps associated with this which is called dysmenorrhoea and is absolutely not normal.

It's something that we didn't really study 20 years ago and are only really making the link with now. These days those patients will be put on the contraceptive pill to regulate their cycle, but I have seen women come in with a 10-year history of very heavy periods who have never been treated.

Those women have suffered and by the time they come to see me they have severe fatigue and exhaustion, but when you go back in their history a key aspect is those very heavy cycles where they would have lost a lot of blood, lost a lot of iron and been pretty much exhausted for one week out of four every month.

This is something that we're tuning into a lot more now, which is great, though it is a shame it didn't happen earlier. In our society, there has been a culture of saying nothing about your cycle, or if you did mention pain, you'd be given some pain relief and advised to use a hot water bottle. Women's pain was very much underappreciated and often brushed off. But we know now that none of that is part of a normal cycle and should be immediately investigated.

Imagine a 12-year-old with painful periods. You would do everything in your power as a parent to make sure your child didn't suffer, perhaps the way you did.

Now, although I have said that girls are getting their periods at 12, it's still very common to not get your first one until you're 16. If you have a 15-year-old who hasn't menstruated yet, don't be alarmed; the span is from 8 to 16.

Our cycles stop at menopause (which is one full year without periods) when we stop ovulating, which is typically around 50 years of age.

A normal menstrual cycle

It is important to know what a normal cycle looks like. Whether you're a young woman starting on her journey, a couple trying to conceive or a woman nearing perimenopause or menopause, knowing what a normal cycle is will be your benchmark for judging whether something may be wrong.

There are four phases:

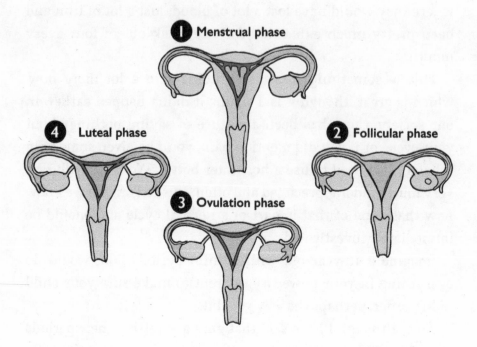

The menstrual phase is where it all starts; although you might see it as the end, it's actually the beginning of your new cycle. It typically lasts from day 1 to day 5 and is when the lining of the uterus is shed through the vagina if pregnancy has not occurred that month.

The follicular phase usually takes place from day 6 to day 14 and is when your oestrogen levels rise, which causes the lining of the uterus (the endometrium) to thicken. At the same time, the FSH causes the follicles in the ovaries to grow and during days 10–14 one of those follicles will produce an ovum or fully mature egg.

Ovulation is the phase that occurs roughly halfway through your cycle on day 14. A sudden rise in LH causes the ovary to release its egg ready for its journey to fertilisation (or not).

The luteal phase lasts from day 15 to day 28 in a typical 28-day cycle. When the egg is released by the ovary it makes its way down through the fallopian tubes and into the uterus. During this time the levels of progesterone rise to help get the uterine lining ready for pregnancy. If the egg is fertilised by a sperm and attaches itself to the uterine wall, pregnancy occurs. If this doesn't happen, oestrogen and progesterone levels drop, the lining of the uterus is shed and we're back to the menstrual phase!

While excessive bleeding and pain that interferes with your life are not normal, there can still be side effects to your menstrual cycle that are. Here are some that you can expect:

- Mood changes
- Difficulty sleeping
- Cravings (often for sugar or carbohydrates)
- Some cramping in your lower back and abdomen
- Bloating
- Breast tenderness
- Acne

There are times when you should speak to your doctor:

- If you haven't started your period by the age of 16
- If your periods stop suddenly
- If you're bleeding for longer than usual
- If your bleeding is heavier than usual
- If you're in a lot of pain
- If you have bleeding between your periods
- If you feel unwell after using tampons
- If you stop taking the pill and your period doesn't return within three months (and you know that you're not pregnant)

- If you have any questions at all. Questions about your body and its well-being are totally normal and should be normalised. If you have a question, ask it – your doctor is there to answer your questions. You never know when a simple question might reveal something about your health, and you'll be glad that you asked.

Changes to your hormones or ovulation may cause a long period. You may notice hormonal changes when you first get your period during puberty or in perimenopause. You may also experience a hormonal imbalance from different health conditions, such as thyroid disorders or polycystic ovary syndrome.

Period pain

Period pain is caused by prostaglandins, which are hormone-like compounds that have a variety of physiological effects including the constriction of blood vessels. High histamine levels also play a role in period pain.

Zinc is a great supplement for period pain and it reduces inflammation and prostaglandins. Magnesium also reduces prostaglandins. You can take an NSAID (non-steroidal anti-inflammatory, e.g. ibuprofen) and sometimes it is necessary to give an oral contraceptive pill or cyclical progesterone therapy.

Precocious puberty

While 12 might sound like a young age to get your first period, there is a condition called precocious puberty that results in it happening even earlier. It's when puberty begins before the age of eight in girls and nine in boys. The cause can't always be found but is sometimes linked to infections, hormone disorders, tumours, brain abnormalities or injuries.

If you're concerned about precocious puberty in your child, you should look out for adult body odour, acne, fast growth, pubic or underarm hair, breast growth and the first period in girls and enlarged testicles and penis, facial hair and a deepening voice in boys. Treatment usually includes medication to delay further development.

Premenstrual syndrome (PMS)

Premenstrual syndrome is a condition that affects women around day 14 and lasts until approximately seven days after menstruation. PMS is the name given to the symptoms that many women experience in the weeks before they get their period each month. Nearly 80% of women report one or more symptoms and if you suffer from it you know all about it.

Unfortunately, PMS was one of those things that women thought they needed to suffer in silence, but of course, we now know that like so much of women's health complaints, that silent suffering is unnecessary.

Ovulation needs a rise in LH to happen, and if the pituitary gland is tired due to hormonal imbalance, you are going to have a knock-on effect due to the stress that's caused as it attempts to raise the hormone. This imbalance is going to result in PMS.

Symptoms

PMS generally starts between 5 and 11 days before your period and goes away or eases once your period begins.

The symptoms occur any time between puberty and menopause, but the most common age is 20 to 30. Stress and overwork exacerbate PMS due to pituitary fatigue, which I've mentioned before. You'll notice that time and time again I will come back to pituitary fatigue as an explanation for conditions you might be experiencing. The importance of minding your body and listening to it when you're tired truly cannot be overstated.

I have met patients with severe PMS and it is a condition that needs more sympathy from the medical profession. For example, when researching this book I read that some doctors feel only women with severe symptoms have true PMS. Fewer than 5% of women get a more severe form of PMS called premenstrual dysmorphic disorder. To dismiss the rest of women who 'only' experience regular PMS is to turn your back on a large percentage of the population.

This is nonsense and if women have symptoms, they have symptoms. As women, we know what suffering is around a menstrual period and how some days and months it is easier to cope and some days are better than others.

My hypothesis on PMS is that you have a tired pituitary caused by heavy periods or anovulatory cycles, which is a menstrual cycle where ovulation doesn't happen. If there is an imbalance between LH and FSH, there is an effect on all the other neurotransmitters at the peripheral nerve–muscle junction – hence the muscle pain, headaches and abdominal bloating (remember, the bowel is a muscle). When there is a hormonal imbalance there is a problem at every nerve–muscle junction.

As a result of the peripheral nerve pain, there is restless sleep, and this exacerbates fatigue and your emotional lability, which is rapid changes to your mood where you might have very strong emotions or feelings (including laughing, crying or temper). Those quick mood changes will be very familiar to a lot of women.

Up to 80% of women report at least one symptom of PMS during their cycle without it affecting them day to day, and between 20% and 32% of women report more severe symptoms that have an impact on their daily life. Symptoms and their severity can change from month to month and can include:

- Sore breasts
- Acne
- Abdominal bloating and pain
- Heavy cravings for sugar or carbohydrates
- Constipation
- Diarrhoea
- Anxiety
- Depression
- Low mood
- Irritability
- Changes in sleep
- Fatigue
- Headaches
- Sadness
- Peripheral nerve pain

Some people find that taking supplements can help with their symptoms. Folic acid and vitamin B6 contribute to healthy nervous function and there is some evidence that magnesium could play a role in reducing cramps and mood swings. I'm a big advocate for looking at your lifestyle and recommend eating a healthy diet, cutting down on sugar and getting some exercise. Sleep and good-quality rest are also really important for reducing PMS.

CASE HISTORY: JULIANNE

Julianne had been suffering from severe PMS since puberty. She was 24 when she was referred to me and had severe migraines, fatigue, IBS, restless legs, and severe muscle tenderness over her biceps on both arms as well as over her trapezius muscles (across her back). Some call this fibromyalgia but I call it peripheral nerve pain as it gives it a scientific basis and is not dismissive of the symptom of pain, which is very severe for a lot of patients.

Her energy levels were very low and her GP had told her she was depressed. However, she knew she was not depressed; she had completed a law degree, had a busy life, didn't feel anxious and was only suffering at certain times of the month. I discovered that she had very heavy periods that lasted seven days and had done since puberty. Her peripheral nerve pain and restless legs were disrupting her sleep. I treated her heavy periods by giving progesterone to correct the luteal phase defect, reducing their length from seven days to three, and also treated her peripheral nerve pain.

I put her on a healthy diet and asked her to omit sugar which she had been craving due to her exhaustion and low cortisol levels. I insisted on the lifestyle changes and asked her to slow down.

Julianne was totally unaware of how well she was doing in life. She was a high achiever and felt that she always had to prove herself, so when I pointed all this out to her, she was amazed. She didn't get a lot of praise at home, so we spoke about self-esteem and self-worth, and I recommended she read *Self Esteem: The Key to Your Child's Future* by the great Irish psychologist Dr Tony Humphreys.

So much of the exhaustion a lot of my patients feel stems from pushing too hard and trying to prove something they don't need to. Julianne was the same, and though I was sad she felt that way, I was happy that she was young, and I could speak to her about it early in her life.

Once we had an insight into what was going on with her health and I sorted out her hormonal problems, she went away to make the lifestyle changes I recommended and work on her self-esteem and we met in the middle. She did well, and I was able to wean her off her medication within six months.

Explaining PMS to your partner

If I had my way, every young man in the country would receive an education in women's health. We know an awful lot about men's health, while they can manage to get through life knowing very little about us at all. If your partner is a man, there is a real benefit to sitting him down and explaining what happens to you each month. Many men haven't the first idea what we go through because they were kept away from the women's part of sex education in school and we have historically been taught to say nothing. This is not normal and it is not fair to men either; they need to know about our hormones so that they can support us at home and in the workplace. We must remember that we are 50% of the population and they are also 50% so it is time for us to work together and for us to insist that we are seen as equal because we know we are equal.

They might roll their eyes and say you're moody, but if you explain the complex hormonal dance that happens in your body each month, they may be surprised you're not in bad form more often!

I find that the best way of doing this is to start with the facts. Explain what happens during a menstrual cycle and how there are different stages that each has different hormonal fluctuations. Then explain what happens each month if you are not pregnant.

I find that if you liken it to the changes they experienced in their bodies at puberty but explain that it happens each and every month, they have a better understanding of the huge shifts you experience. Tell them that there are times of the month when you need more rest and some peace. Start with periods and PMS, then, as the years go by, explain perimenopause and menopause.

Explain things clearly and concisely and don't be embarrassed; it's all part of a normal healthy life!

When I was giving a lecture on hormonal health with Lorraine Keane as MC, I was delighted when she told me that her 18-year-old daughter Emelia had said to her boyfriend that she was in bad form due to having PMS. Wasn't that music to my ears? She had heard Lorraine and me talking so much about hormonal health and PMS that it normalised discussing it with her partner.

Cravings and your period

A lot of women have cravings around the time of their period that they don't experience at any other time. Those cravings usually involve chocolate, sugar or carbohydrates and there is a good scientific reason for them.

The hormonal changes your body goes through during your period, especially the fluctuating levels of oestrogen and progesterone, make your body think it needs these sweet or stodgy treats. You experience a little boost of serotonin, the happy hormone, when you eat those types of foods around your period.

The cravings usually happen around the same time that you might experience other premenstrual symptoms like PMS, headaches or bloating and so that little boost of serotonin is very welcome.

A treat every so often is fine – I do believe in everything in moderation – but if you consume too much of that kind of food it will only make you feel worse in the long run. I always advise that people try to get their boost of happy hormones in another way. Exercise, spending time with loved ones or making your own healthier versions of your favourite snacks will all make you feel better without a sugar hangover.

Remember that if you do indulge, make sure not to do it too close to bedtime as it will disrupt your sleep. If you don't get good sleep, you'll only feel worse the next day and your hormonal vortex will be out of balance.

Oligomenorrhoea and amenorrhoea

Oligomenorrhoea is when you have infrequent periods. These usually have a cycle length of more than 35 days or fewer than nine menstrual cycles a year.

Amenorrhoea is the name for absent periods and there are two types, primary and secondary. **Primary amenorrhoea** is when a young girl doesn't start her period, and this will usually cause a GP to send her for an assessment with a paediatric consultant. **Secondary amenorrhoea** is where you have previously had a menstrual cycle which stops without explanation (such as pregnancy).

For an official diagnosis of amenorrhoea, your period will have been absent for six months. A one-off missed period isn't of great concern, although, as I always say, listen to your body and if you feel there's a bigger issue, speak to your doctor.

There are a couple of obvious causes of amenorrhoea that are easy to rule out. The first is pregnancy and the second is breastfeeding. Women who exclusively breastfeed often see a delay in their periods returning after they have given birth.

Once those two causes are ruled out there are some other things to look out for. Thyroid disease, premature ovarian failure (which we used to call early menopause) and polycystic ovary syndrome can all be causes of amenorrhoea.

A prolactin imbalance is another cause and is one that I see in my clinic. Prolactin is a hormone that comes from our pituitary gland and is vital for our reproductive health. Anything that increases prolactin can disrupt the normal menstrual cycle.

Some medicines (like some anti-nausea drugs and some anti-psychotic medications) can increase your prolactin levels and may also disrupt your menstrual cycle.

Stress can also increase your prolactin levels, which might have a knock-on effect on your cycle. You already know how I feel about too much stress in your life and how it affects almost everything in your body. Your menstrual cycle is no different, as it too is controlled by a delicate balance of hormones.

If there is a change in your cycle and your periods stop, you should speak to your doctor. They will need to check your thyroid function, prolactin levels and LH and FSH levels as well as your oestrogen and testosterone levels. You may also need to have an ultrasound of your pelvis to rule out ovarian cysts.

Causes of amenorrhoea

- Pregnancy
- Breastfeeding
- Thyroid disease
- Polycystic ovary syndrome
- High prolactin – whether caused by a prolactinoma (a non-cancerous tumour of the pituitary gland), psychological stress or medication
- Premature ovarian failure

Menorrhagia

This is the medical term for heavy or prolonged periods.

Every woman's cycle is different and what is heavy for one woman may not be for another, but again, it's important to know what is normal and what is not.

A normal period is a blood volume of less than 80ml but it's very difficult to know the exact amount of blood you're losing, so instead, we talk about how often you soak through one sanitary pad or tampon. If you need to change protection every hour, if you need to wake during the night to change your pad, if you are passing clots larger than a 50-cent piece, if you are bleeding for more than a week or if you are very tired or find yourself short of breath, you may have menorrhagia.

The most common cause of it is those anovulatory cycles I mentioned in the section on PMS.

In a normal cycle, the release of an egg tells the body to produce progesterone, which is the hormone responsible for keeping periods regular. If no egg is released in a cycle and your body doesn't produce that progesterone, it can cause heavy bleeding.

There are several things that can contribute to a hormonal imbalance that results in menorrhagia, including polycystic ovary syndrome, obesity, insulin resistance and thyroid problems.

Teenage girls are especially prone to having anovulatory cycles in the first year of their period and often experience heavy bleeding just as they're starting their menstrual journey.

Heavy bleeding can put you at risk of blood loss, anaemia or low iron, which is why it's important for women to report heavy or prolonged bleeding to their doctor.

You might feel excessively tired or weak and you might have pale skin. In very severe cases there may be breathlessness because there aren't enough red blood cells in your body to deliver oxygen to your lungs. Sometimes all this happens at such a slow and steady pace that women may not notice the symptoms coming on and don't go to see the doctor until things are quite bad.

A number of things can cause heavy bleeding including fibroids, which are benign growths in the uterus, and adenomyosis, which is when the cells that should be in the lining of the uterus are infiltrating the muscular part of the uterus. Polyps, which are small benign growths in the lining of the uterus, can also cause prolonged, heavy bleeding.

Bleeding disorders, blood clotting diseases and an underactive thyroid can also be causes and your doctor might do a blood test to rule those out. Heavy bleeding is a well-known side effect of using a copper coil or non-hormonal intrauterine device. If that happens, your doctor can suggest alternative contraceptive options.

If you're postmenopausal and are experiencing bleeding, you should immediately speak to your doctor. Heavy bleeding can also be a symptom of endometrial cancer, which is more common in older women.

Treatments for menorrhagia include progesterone, which often restores more regular bleeding. Some patients may need the Mirena, or hormonal, coil, which has a slow release of progesterone.

Causes of menorrhagia

- Fibroids
- Adenomyosis (a condition where the endometrial tissue grows into the muscular wall of the uterus)
- Bleeding disorders
- Underactive thyroid

- Blood thinning medicines
- Endometritis (inflammation of the lining of the uterus)
- Pelvic inflammatory disease
- Copper coil
- Endometrial cancer

CASE HISTORY: ANNE

Anne was 24 when she came to see me complaining of severe fatigue, muscle pain and not sleeping. She had started puberty at 12 and had periods that lasted seven days and came with severe cramps. She was in college studying law and doing well.

I could see a few issues. She had been having seven-day periods for 12 years and nothing had been done to treat them. That would exhaust anyone's pituitary gland, and no one had even investigated the extreme pain that she was in each month.

She was also pushing herself very hard in college and was doing more than her body could cope with. I treated her physical pain and her lengthy periods and she committed to pacing herself and listening to her body.

Each patient is different but I treated her period problems by giving her progesterone in the luteal phase. This helped with pain and bleeding. With this kind of patient, I am trying to reset the rhythm of the menstrual cycle. Often you only need to be on the medication for six months.

I told Anne that if her hormonal system was already in flux at 24, in another 10 years she could be very unwell.

She did well with treatment and sent me a card when she had her first baby many years later.

I do not doubt that if we hadn't got to the root of her problem at 24, things would have been very different when it came time to start her family.

CHAPTER FOUR
Fertility

Deciding to have a baby can be the most joyous and nerve-wracking time in a couple's lives. For a lot of women and couples, once the decision is made, things happen very smoothly, and pregnancy occurs within a few months.

For others, it takes time. I know that the longer the trying goes on the more nervous and stressed a woman can become.

There are things that you can do to prepare for pregnancy and try to make the journey to becoming pregnant as smooth as you can. First and foremost, look at your lifestyle. It sounds very simplistic but make sure you have a healthy diet, don't smoke or be around smokers and cut your alcohol consumption – and that goes for both men and women.

I'm adamant that men take an active role in trying to conceive and don't lay all the pressure at the feet of women. Most men nowadays are very willing to be involved and are very supportive, which is the way it should be, and they enjoy the journey with their partner.

Take folic acid and vitamin D and make sure you're getting a sensible amount of exercise. There is evidence now that vitamin D reduces the risk of gestational diabetes and pre-eclampsia. Men should also take vitamin C and make sure that their diet incorporates zinc and selenium – both can improve sperm quality.

If either of you has any existing medical conditions, it's a good idea to speak to your doctors about any medications you might be on – some of them can interfere with conception so it's always wise to double-check.

Previous abdominal surgeries can sometimes result in internal scarring which might block the fallopian tubes, so that is something to bear in mind. Men who have had mumps orchitis (mumps that affected the testicles) or any history of testicular trauma may also have difficulty conceiving.

Forewarned is forearmed and the more information you can give your doctors the better. Remember when I said that patient history is vital? Well, you're the only one who can tell your specialist that you had your appendix out when you were 17 or that your partner had a sporting injury in his 20s. We really do appreciate *all* the information you can give us.

It's important too to be able to give your doctor a comprehensive overview of your menstrual cycle. One of the reasons I'm so passionate about women understanding what normal periods are is because if you end up having difficulty conceiving you will be able to explain your cycle in detail.

If a patient comes to me and immediately says she has a six-day period that's very heavy with a moderate amount of pain or she has a 33-day, quite unpredictable cycle, I know what we're dealing with and how to proceed.

Fertility

So, let's talk about fertility.

When you know your menstrual cycle, you increase your chances of getting pregnant. Your cycle begins, and not ends as many believe, with the first day of your period. Your cycle has four phases and the first begins on the first day of bleeding.

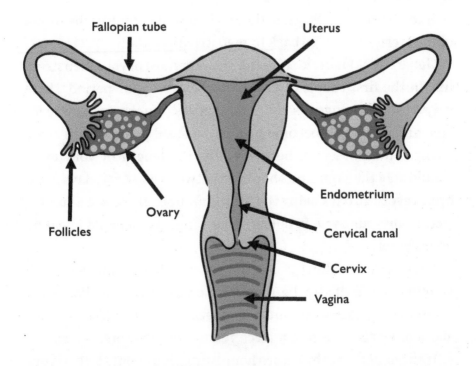

The four phases are the menstrual phase (bleeding); the follicular phase (before the release of the egg); the ovulatory phase (the release of the egg); and the luteal phase (after the release of the egg).

The first half of the menstrual cycle is dominated by FSH coming from the pituitary gland. This hormone stimulates the ovaries to develop follicles that contain eggs. Those follicles produce rising levels of oestrogen that thickens the lining of the uterus.

In the middle of the cycle, the pituitary gland releases a spike of LH that causes the egg to be released from the follicle, and that's ovulation. The egg travels from the ovary to the uterus via the fallopian tubes. If the egg is then fertilised by sperm it will create an embryo which will travel down the fallopian tubes into the uterus, and that's pregnancy.

If there is no fertilisation, there will be a shedding of the lining of the uterus and we're back to menstruation again.

Generally, your cycle stays the same for most of your menstrual life. In the first couple of years after you get your period, there may be some changes as your body settles into the right cycle for you, and when you become perimenopausal you may see some changes to your cycle, but generally, the length of your cycle should stay the same and should be between 28 and 35 days (with cycles every 28 days being the most common). If you see a sudden change or your cycle is outside that range, you should speak to your doctor.

Your cycle shouldn't cause you any trouble or interfere with your daily life. It can be annoying or inconvenient but there shouldn't be excess amounts of bleeding that you're worried about or levels of pain that force you to cancel events.

If either of those things are happening, you should talk to your doctor, regardless of whether you're planning a family.

Trying to conceive

Ovulation usually occurs between days 11 and 21 of your cycle and is different for everyone, which is why listening to your body is important. You might notice that you get an increase in cervical mucus and discharge around that time; this is your body's way of helping sperm get to your egg more easily. However, most women ovulate around day 14 of their cycle.

Amazingly, women are born with between one million and two million eggs, though we release only about 300 or 400 in our lifetime. You usually release just one egg each month, which is why timing is so important if you wish to conceive.

If the egg isn't fertilised within 24 hours of leaving the ovary it dissolves, but sperm can live for about three to five days, so generally the best chance of pregnancy is when you have sex one or two days before ovulation.

It takes about 24 hours for a sperm to fertilise an egg and once it has done so the form of the egg changes so that no other sperm can get in. At the very moment of fertilisation, the baby's genetic make-up is complete – isn't nature fascinating?

Things move fast from this point onwards. The egg starts growing and dividing into many cells. About three or four days after fertilisation it leaves the fallopian tubes and enters the uterus. Once it gets there it attaches to the lining called the endometrium, and this is implantation.

After about a week the hormone HCG (human chorionic gonadotropin) can be found in the mother's blood. This is what shows up in a blood or urine pregnancy test.

When the egg attaches to the uterus, some of the cells become the placenta and some become the embryo. The heart starts beating at about five weeks and the brain and spinal cord begin to form. At about the eight-week mark, the embryo becomes a foetus.

Infertility

When you're trying to conceive and it isn't happening, it is heartbreaking. Every month you're not pregnant can feel like a failure and over time you feel upset, anxious and more stressed. We need to stop asking couples if they have any news, as a lot of those couples are trying hard to get pregnant and could well do without inquisitive people putting more pressure on them.

Infertility is a lot more common than people realise, but I know that telling a woman that can be of little comfort. Infertility is defined as not being able to get pregnant despite trying for at least a year, or six months if you're over 35, though your doctor may evaluate you sooner if you have risk factors such as an irregular cycle, endometriosis or pelvic inflammatory disease. Pelvic inflammatory disease can cause salpingitis, which is an inflammation of the fallopian tubes. This is usually caused by endometriosis, adhesions or a sexually transmitted infection.

Infertility can result from problems with the woman's reproductive system, the man's sperm production or a combination of the two together.

The World Health Organization (WHO) performed a large multinational study to determine gender distribution and infertility causes. In 37% of infertile couples, female infertility was the cause; in 35% of infertile couples, both male and female causes were identified; and in 8% of infertile couples, there was male factor infertility. In the remaining 20% of couples, no cause could be identified, which is known as unexplained infertility.

In the same study, the most common identifiable factors of female infertility were as follows:

- Ovulatory disorders – 25%
- Endometriosis – 15%
- Pelvic adhesions – 12%
- Tubal blockage – 11%
- Other tubal/uterine abnormalities – 11%
- Hyperprolactinemia – 7%

It is important to realise that male factor infertility represents a substantial portion of the identifiable factors causing infertility.

Infertility can also be caused by abnormalities of the cervix, polyps in the uterus or the shape of the uterus (a bicornate uterus). There can also be fibroids, which are benign cysts that can sometimes block the fallopian tubes or stop a fertilised egg implanting successfully.

A woman might start investigations with a gynaecologist, who will run some physical tests before they refer her to an endocrinologist like me.

Tests that you might have when experiencing infertility

- Day 21 progesterone test to see if ovulation has occurred. For women who don't have a 28-day cycle, the test can be done seven days before their expected period.
- A day 3 FSH test.
- Thyroid function tests.
- Testosterone levels check.
- Prolactin levels check.
- AMH (anti-mullerian hormone) blood test.
- STI check.

- A laparoscopy and dye test to check that your fallopian tubes are clear. This is a day-case keyhole surgery done by a gynaecologist to assess fallopian tube health. A dye is injected through the tubes to make sure that they're open.
- A transvaginal (internal) ultrasound of the pelvis.
- A hysterosalpingogram, which is a specialised scan and a less invasive way of assessing the health of the fallopian tubes.
- Semen analysis to check the health, shape, motility (movement) and number of sperm.

Anovulation

One of the main reasons a woman may not become pregnant is because she is not ovulating. Lots of women still have periods without ovulating and so you may not know that it is happening. This can be caused by a number of things.

Premature ovarian failure is an autoimmune condition where the immune system attacks the ovaries; it is sometimes called early menopause. If you have this condition your ovaries will stop working and your periods will end before the age of 40.

Hyperprolactinaemia is when you have too much prolactin which interferes with ovulation. Prolactin levels are high in women who are pregnant or have just given birth (it controls milk production), but if it is high before you conceive it can cause infertility.

Hyperthyroidism and **hypothyroidism** can also interfere with the menstrual cycle and your fertility.

Polycystic ovary syndrome (PCOS)

Polycystic ovary syndrome is a cause of infertility in women. It is an endocrinopathy, which means a disease of the endocrine gland. Simply put, it is a hormonal problem.

It's thought to be one of the most common forms of endocrinopathy in women, affecting between 5% and 10% of women around the world. PCOS affects women of reproductive age. The women affected by it have multiple cysts on their ovaries. It's very important to remember, however, that if you have cysts on your ovaries, that doesn't necessarily mean that you have PCOS. Ovarian cysts and PCOS are two very different things.

Hormonal changes are an important part of a PCOS diagnosis.

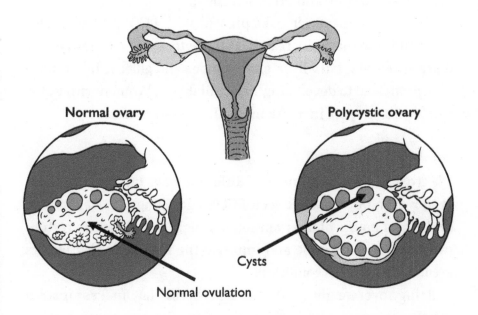

Normal ovary

Polycystic ovary

Cysts

Normal ovulation

The symptoms of PCOS include oligomenorrhoea (infrequent periods), excess hair on the upper lip, chin, neck, chest and abdomen, acne, difficulty conceiving and weight gain.

According to the Rotterdam Criteria, PCOS is defined by the presence of two or three of the following: irregular periods; hyperandrogenism; polycystic ovaries with greater than 12 follicles measuring 2–9mm in diameter and an ovarian volume of greater than 10ml in at least one ovary.

Clinically, we characterise PCOS by oligomenorrhoea and hyperandrogenism. Androgens are your sex hormones and in PCOS you have an excess of them, hence hyperandrogenism.

One of the first signs that point women towards a diagnosis of PCOS is infrequent periods. With PCOS, the menstrual cycle is disrupted. Multiple small follicles accumulate on the ovary, but none of them develops to a size large enough to trigger ovulation. This results in an imbalance between the reproductive hormones, LH, FSH, oestrogen and progesterone.

There are some other risks present with PCOS. Women with the condition have increased risk factors for cardiovascular disease, obesity, fatty liver, sleep apnoea and glucose intolerance which can lead to developing Type 2 diabetes. Women with PCOS can have a 50–70% increase in insulin resistance.

Treating PCOS

We treat PCOS in a number of different ways but because there is shown to be a link between PCOS and being overweight, one of the first points of intervention is weight loss. This can restore ovulation in your cycle and improve the metabolic risk factors associated with the condition.

Being overweight and having excess fat makes insulin resistance worse and high levels of insulin can cause further weight gain, so you can see how it is a vicious circle.

I know that having weight loss suggested as a treatment for PCOS can be disheartening, especially when any weight gain happened because you have the syndrome. I also know that losing it can be easier said than done, but it is an excellent first-line intervention.

Women with PCOS are often pointed towards anti-inflammatory diets to help manage their weight and symptoms. I am a big believer in moderation and in the Mediterranean diet. Be sure to include lots of fibre, fish and fresh, vibrantly coloured vegetables on your plate.

PCOS can develop into high cholesterol, heart disease, high blood pressure and Type 2 diabetes, so making those changes to the diet is a great first step. It's the diet we should all be aiming for, regardless of any hormonal conditions we may have.

Then we use a combination of different medications to combat the other symptoms. Metformin makes the body more sensitive to insulin and reduces insulin resistance. Other treatments combat excess androgens.

Decreased menstrual periods in PCOS means that there is a build-up of the lining of the uterus, which can put women at increased risk of endometrial cancer, so one of the benefits of prescribing the oral contraceptive pill is that there can be a monthly withdrawal bleed to prevent that build-up of the endometrium.

If a patient is trying to become pregnant, I would help her to lose weight and to become pregnant by giving her a high dose of FSH to stimulate ovulation. Losing weight is key and helping sort out the hormonal imbalance in PCOS helps these women to do this.

Exercise is a very good way of improving insulin sensitivity as it builds muscle and improves glucose uptake into cells.

Note that finding polycystic ovaries characteristic of PCOS via ultrasound is unlikely to occur in your 40s as you have fewer eggs or follicles at this age.

CASE HISTORY: DEIRDRE

At 44, Deirdre's periods became irregular and stopped for six months. She had always had seven-day cycles so she thought she was in menopause.

We did blood tests. Her FSH was in the non-menopausal range. A pelvic ultrasound showed a thickened uterine lining and normal ovaries. She also had facial hair, acne and excess androgens in her blood. I tested her for insulin resistance and she had some. This combination of irregular periods, facial hair, thickened uterine lining, weight gain and insulin resistance is typical of PCOS.

I worked to reverse her insulin resistance with diet and Metformin and gave her cyclical progesterone therapy to thin her uterine lining and restore ovulation. She did very well.

Endometriosis

Endometriosis is an area where a lot more research needs to be done. Women with this painful condition have suffered dreadfully over the years, waiting a long time for a diagnosis and their symptoms and pain are simply not taken seriously by medical professionals. Although we know more about endometriosis than we've ever known before, a lot more needs to be done and it is a shame that it has taken this long for adequate research to be carried out into this condition that has caused so much suffering to so many women.

The endometrium is the lining of the uterus and patients with endometriosis have endometrial cells growing outside their uterus. When endometrial-like tissue grows outside the uterus it can cause scar tissue, also called adhesions, which can fuse the organs and create connections between them that would not normally be there. This can lead to severe discomfort and pain, but the condition can also cause bloating, digestive problems, bleeding between periods, painful periods, painful intercourse, difficulty conceiving and infertility.

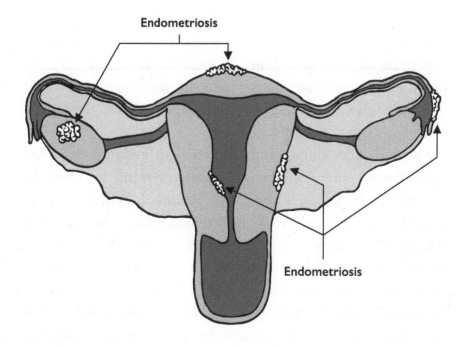

The most common places that endometriosis occurs are the ovaries, the fallopian tubes and the bowel but it can occur in any part of the body.

Endometriosis cannot be diagnosed with blood tests or scans; it often takes a surgical procedure to diagnose it. The reluctance of a lot of doctors to subject patients to unnecessary surgery can be one of the causes of delay in diagnosis. Hormones, especially oestrogen and progesterone, play a major role in endometriosis. The growth and symptoms of endometrial cells are connected to changes in these hormones: low levels of progesterone plus increased oestrogen levels are thought to simultaneously play a role.

Endometriosis is considered an oestrogen-dependent condition. The elevated oestrogen levels that occur with endometriosis trigger inflammation and the growth of endometrial cells in the body. Progesterone also plays a role in preventing the excess growth of endometrial cells.

Patients with endometriosis have imbalanced levels of oestrogen and progesterone in their bodies. Many of the treatments involve ways of rebalancing these levels. Reducing oestrogen levels can help relieve symptoms and prevent the further growth of endometrial cells.

Research also shows that women with endometriosis and adenomyosis (where endometrial tissue grows into the muscular wall of the uterus) have abnormal immune function including altered levels and behaviour of immune cells, especially mast cells (which control immune responses), and higher levels of autoantibodies (which attack the body's tissue) and inflammatory cytokines (which can lead to inflammatory diseases). I am fascinated by the research that shows that a disruption in your gut microbiome (which we will discuss later) can contribute to endometriosis and I am looking forward to the day when probiotic treatments will help this very painful condition. These treatments have already been effective in treating endometriosis in humans and animals but more research is needed.

Research also suggests that with the immune dysfunction of endometriosis and adenomyosis, the immune system does not remove lesions but instead promotes their growth with inflammatory cytokines. It has also been suggested that an underlying problem with the gut microbiome and intestinal permeability contributes directly to inflammation and adenomyosis. This has been supported by a review study that linked endometriosis with an imbalance of gut bacteria. According to the bacterial contamination hypothesis of endometriosis, women with endometriosis have intestinal permeability, which causes gut bacteria to enter the pelvic cavity and release toxins that promote immune dysfunction.

Factors that can put you at higher risk of developing endometriosis

- Family history of endometriosis.
- The age at which you start your periods. People who begin menstruating before 11 are at higher risk.
- The length of your menstrual cycle and the duration of flow.

People who experience symptoms of endometriosis may have the following:

- Very painful periods
- Abdominal pain or back pain during periods
- Pain during sex
- Heavy bleeding during periods
- Infertility
- Painful bowel movements

Your menstrual cycle is driven by fluctuations in hormone levels, especially oestrogen and progesterone. An imbalance of hormone levels in your body can also contribute to fatigue, a common endometriosis symptom. A small qualitative study in 2020 found that the vast majority of females living with moderate to severe endometriosis experience fatigue.

I've seen patients who have suffered terribly with endometriosis and I believe that the earlier we can get to it the better. That's why we must listen to young women when they're talking about their menstrual health, and they have to be believed when it comes to pain levels and other symptoms. There is no connection between the symptoms and the severity. Some people may only have a few patches of endometriosis but still experience severe pain.

Treatments for endometriosis

The treatment involves the regulation of oestrogen and progesterone levels. Each woman with endometriosis is different and so each treatment plan will be different. There is no outright cure for the disease, but treatment can help to ease symptoms and pain levels.

Treatments include:

- Painkillers.
- Contraceptives – the combined oral contraceptive pill or progesterone-containing coils like Mirena. Gonadotrophin-releasing hormones are also used to stop the hormones that cause the menstrual cycle. This puts your reproductive system on hold as a way to relieve pain. Utrogestan works in much the same way as progesterone but has fewer side effects.
- Antihistamine medication can relieve symptoms for some women because of the role histamine and mast cell activation play in the development of endometriosis.

Antihistamines can also lighten the blood flow. This area needs more research.

- Surgery to remove lesions and endometrial tissue – endometrial ablation is a procedure that surgically destroys the lining of the uterus with the goal of reducing menstrual flow. Uterine artery embolisation attempts to shrink adenomyosis by cutting off its blood supply. The procedure carries a higher risk of complications for adenomyosis than for fibroids.
- Operations to remove parts of or all of the organs affected by the disease, such as a hysterectomy, which is the surgical removal of the uterus. Hysterectomy is the last step but for some, it is the right choice, especially if they are still suffering dreadfully despite a variety of other treatments. If your ovaries are removed, and you go into surgical menopause, you should go on HRT (hormone replacement therapy). Discuss this with your doctor, who will determine what treatment is best and safe for you.
- Antimicrobial and probiotic treatment and research are ongoing in this area.

I really feel for women who are living with this condition. I know a lot of them feel they have been abandoned and left to manage on their own and that's not okay. The education of doctors and young women is key to treating endometriosis as well as further research into causes and treatment.

Chronic fatigue

We've already talked about chronic fatigue in Chapter Two, but it is a big factor in infertility.

I believe there's almost always an answer for unexplained infertility. That's not to say that there can definitely be a happy outcome every single time, but there is an answer and I believe that couples deserve more than to be told there is no explanation for their infertility. In my experience, the unknown is usually a hormonal imbalance and very often it's pituitary fatigue or a thyroid issue.

For me, it all goes back to taking a proper history. If you really listen to a woman, you'll be able to determine where the problems lie. Symptoms and histories are usually very typical and if you listen, you'll find the key. Often, complete exhaustion is the root cause. So many women are trying to do too much at work, at home, with exercise, with friendships and with socialising. Some things in that scenario have to give. As a society, and particularly as women, we have to learn how to prioritise rest.

It's not always easy, especially when you're trying to conceive and that contributes to your stress levels. We know that stress is bad for our hormonal health, and while it can be very hard to be told, 'if you relax it will happen', there is actual science behind that.

High cortisol and adrenaline levels affect the functioning of the master control gland, the pituitary gland. In order to function properly, the master control gland has to be recharged. It's like your phone that needs to be plugged in at night. Your hormones can't do their job of positive and negative feedback if they're not rested and recharged. There's so much going on and being driven by hormones every millisecond of the day, this complex system needs to be looked after. Running on empty is not an option for your hormonal health.

You will laugh at me now when I say this, but one of the things that I always prescribe is a cleaner! I know this is a luxury so, even if you can't get one, I hope it makes you hear what I'm saying about not doing everything yourself. Partners, in my experience, are almost always brilliant the minute a woman says she's pregnant. Feet go up and they're treated like a delicate package. But what about the months before that? I think every relationship should be 100% equal with household chores divided up and not left to one person all the time. If for some reason, this isn't happening, as soon as you decide to try to have a baby you should be getting rest, getting help and being minded. The months when you are trying to conceive are very important.

Infertility in men

Historically, if there was an issue with infertility, a woman was automatically assumed to be the problem.

It is poor practice to put a woman through a whole range of invasive testing before checking a man's sperm sample. It's such an easy thing to do and I would much rather that is done first as, if there is a reduction in sperm or even no sperm, it's easy to deal with and saves putting the woman through invasive testing.

In the past, it was not uncommon for a woman to be fully investigated without any thought of the man. This included a laparoscopy, which is an invasive procedure where dye is injected into the woman's fallopian tubes to check they are working correctly.

Thankfully, a semen sample check is now one of the first tests to be done when a couple presents with infertility. We check the semen motility, quantity and shape. Semen quality can be improved with selenium and zinc. Some men may have acquired the mumps virus, which reduces the sperm count significantly, so it is important to rule this out.

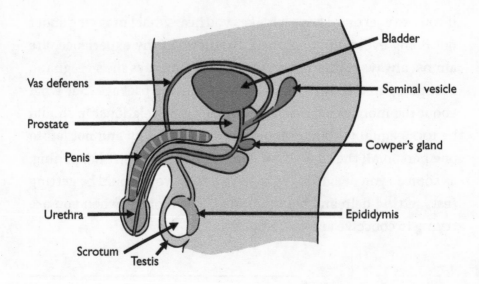

There are some quite common and straightforward causes of male infertility. Lack of semen, poor-quality semen and varicose veins that can affect sperm production are three of the biggest issues. There may also be blockages in the testicles, damage to them from injuries or traumas, or abnormal sperm production due to undescended testes.

Diabetes, HIV, chemotherapy and radiation can also affect sperm quality. Lifestyle factors such as smoking, excess alcohol, marijuana, anabolic steroids and using hot tubs or saunas too frequently can also be a reason for poor-quality sperm.

Men can take an active role in the preparation for conception by improving their overall health, diet and well-being.

Age

One of the things we need to change in society is the messaging around men's fertility and age. Women are very aware of the age limits on their ability to have a child. It's something we hear about time and time again and it puts a lot of pressure on women when it comes to finding a partner they might like to start a family with, but we never talk about age with regard to men. There's a great joke around Mick Jagger and Rod Stewart, who both became fathers for the eighth time at the ages of 73 and 66 respectively, and the virility of the older man. However, when men reach about 50, the quality of their sperm is far lower than they might ever imagine.

In a study conducted by the Centre for Reproductive and Genetic Health in London, it was found that nearly half the male participants in the study under 35 were able to successfully fertilise an egg. For those aged 36–40, that number dropped to 42% and it went down to just 35% for those aged 41–45.

As well as the ability to fertilise, men over the age of 45 have a higher chance of DNA fragmentation, which means a higher risk of genetic damage in the foetus. Women are made very aware of the higher incidence of genetic problems as they get older and have wrongly been made to feel at fault when a couple does not get pregnant, as well as burdened with the fact that being older can cause genetic abnormalities. We now know that the cause of these is just as likely to be a man's issue as a woman's. This is an important fact to know when couples are trying to conceive.

I remember a very frustrated female patient who came to see me. She was 38 and her husband was 46 when she visited the clinic. She was anxious to start a family and didn't want to leave it much longer, aware of the potential issues that come with being an older mum.

Her husband wanted to wait for another five years. He was quite alarmed when I informed him that he did not have that time and that from now on his sperm took on the risk of DNA fragmentation. His wife was thrilled as she was tired of his attitude, and thankfully, they went on to have two very beautiful healthy children.

The message in society needs to change. Women in their 30s are made out to be baby crazy and it's unfair. Men think they have all the time in the world, but they do not.

Also, women should never be called geriatric mothers! This naming and shaming needs to stop in society. A child is a miracle, and if a woman in her late 30s or early 40s wants to have a child she should most certainly not be made to feel embarrassed about her age.

Responsibility for contraception

The responsibility for contraception has always been something that has fallen to women. We were taught, and still teach girls, that if we want to make sure we're protected we must protect ourselves. We've been told that men can't be trusted to take a contraceptive pill and that many will try to avoid other methods of contraception if at all possible. We're letting them off the hook for something that is at least half their responsibility. It is not good enough and we must change that messaging in society.

Even in long-lasting, loving relationships, the burden falls on women, and they can end up taking hormonal contraception even long after their family is complete.

In my time in medicine, I have seen large numbers of women getting tubal ligations as a permanent means of contraception without realising the issue they face afterwards. This is major surgery, and you are at risk of getting early menopause after it. Tubal ligation is a type of permanent birth control where the fallopian tubes are permanently blocked, clipped or removed. Doing this prevents sperm from fertilising an egg.

Having surgery of this kind can cause damage to your bowel or bladder. After the procedure, you can have a decline in oestrogen and progesterone, and I have seen it lead to early menopause. In 2015, there were 450 tubal ligations carried out in Ireland.

Conversely, a male vasectomy is a simple procedure that can be done during a lunch hour with pain that is managed by over-the-counter painkillers. There are few to no side effects. Which do you think is the more sensible option? The one that needs a general anaesthetic or the one that needs a couple of paracetamol?

I always try to suggest that anyone who is thinking about tubal ligation as a method of contraception should consider a vasectomy for their partner instead. There are no adverse effects on the man's health and it also means that the woman who has carried the pregnancies and quite frankly has done enough in the area of family planning already, does not have the burden of worrying about a future pregnancy but also is not taking hormonal treatment that may have an adverse long-term risk for her health.

CASE HISTORY: BREDA

Breda came to see me when she was 32. She had had a tubal ligation and was in early menopause as a result. She was finding it very hard to cope with her menopausal symptoms while looking after a new baby who was just six weeks old. She also had two other children under four at home.

Her consultant knew that this was to be her last baby and because she was having a caesarean section, they suggested she have a tubal ligation. She did not know that early menopause was a potential complication.

The literature suggests that menopause is not a risk, but I can tell you after 20 years of clinical experience that it most definitely is and I caution all my patients about it.

CASE HISTORY: LAUREN

Sometimes I am astonished by the lengths to which women will go to protect their husband's feelings with little or no regard for their own. Lauren was a case in point.

She was a lovely young woman who came to see me after having her fourth child for advice about contraception. She had had problems with the Mirena coil previously and she could not take the oral contraceptive pill as she suffered from severe migraine. The progesterone-only pill also did not suit her.

I spoke to her about the possibility of her husband having a vasectomy, but she was concerned for her husband in case their marriage failed, and he met someone else with whom he might want to have a child. I was speechless. This was a fabulous young woman whose only concern was for a fictional future that her husband may find himself in and not for her own well-being. I asked her how she'd feel if one of her four girls came to her in 30 years' time and said the same thing after she'd given birth to four children. Lauren broke down and could see what I was trying to point out to her.

Her self-esteem was so low that she was not valuing herself or her contribution to the relationship. You might think this is a case from the start of my career but this happened in 2020. Imagine that!

Women are still so conditioned to be responsible for family planning and for their husbands' feelings that they will put their health at risk.

Lauren spoke to her husband, and he agreed to have the procedure. Her concern for his future was all in her head. He was fine.

CASE HISTORY: VICTORIA

Victoria had completed her family when she came in to talk to me. She was a poorly controlled diabetic who had had four children, each by caesarean section.

She had already been advised not to have any more children and I reiterated that to her at our consultation. Since she was a diabetic, I didn't want to risk the added complication of early menopause. I had given her literature on vasectomies a year before this visit and had asked her to have a conversation with her husband about it. At this visit, I spoke to her about it again and her only reply was to say 'What if he meets someone else and wants more children?'

This beautiful woman in front of me was worried about her husband when she had four small children and a condition that was very hard to manage during pregnancy. I was so upset for her.

As I have said, I am totally against tubal ligation as I have seen too many instances of premature menopause following it and so I warn all my patients not to have it. This is an area where we need very large studies. I am personally convinced we should not be doing tubal ligations at all.

I would love to see a public information campaign around vasectomy and to normalise it as a method of contraception. Family planning should and must be a two-person responsibility. If you have carried the babies, you have done your part.

Miscarriage

First, I want to say that if you have experienced a miscarriage, I'm very sorry. It's common, as I'm sure you're tired of hearing, but that doesn't make it any easier for you or your partner.

People will say lots of things to you, hoping that it might help. Things like, 'Well, at least you can get pregnant', 'Thank God it was early on' or 'Isn't it great you've already one at home to mind?' People mean well and often don't know what to say. But loss is loss and it's very hard. There's disappointment and grief that sometimes you feel you're not able to share, which I would very much like to see change.

Often, because one in five pregnancies does sadly end in miscarriage, you may not get to attend the recurrent miscarriage clinic until you have had three losses. That's very tough because of course you want answers. Even when you do get there you may not be spoken to about hormones, so it's important to know that you can be referred to an endocrinologist or gynaecologist.

We should speak about what miscarriage is and what happens. It is defined as a spontaneous loss of a pregnancy before the 20th week. Although about one in five pregnancies ends in miscarriage, the real figure may be a lot higher because they can occur very early in pregnancy, before you might even know you're pregnant.

Most women who experience miscarriage do so in the first trimester of pregnancy, that's before the 12th week. Miscarriages after that only account for between 1% and 5% of losses.

Miscarriages happen because the foetus isn't growing as expected. You will sometimes hear that at a scan appointment when they say that it is measuring 'behind'. About half of all miscarriages are associated with chromosomal issues, where there are either extra chromosomes or missing ones. Most of the time, those chromosomal problems happen by chance and not because of problems with the parents. If you have three or more miscarriages, you and your partner will be offered chromosomal screening to rule that out.

Chromosome problems can lead to:

- A molar pregnancy – both sets of chromosomes come from the father and there is abnormal growth of the placenta. There is usually no foetal development. A partial molar pregnancy happens when there are two sets of chromosomes from the father, but the mother's chromosomes are there too. This is usually associated with an abnormal placenta and foetus.
- A blighted ovum – this happens when no embryo forms.
- Intrauterine foetal demise – this is when an embryo forms but stops developing and dies before there are any symptoms of pregnancy loss. Intrauterine foetal demise is also called stillbirth and happens after the 20th week of pregnancy.

There are other things that can cause miscarriage too. Infection, improper implantation of your fertilised egg, an incompetent cervix (this involves weak cervical tissue), uterine abnormalities, the age of the woman and hormone irregularities can all be contributory factors.

Uterine abnormalities can often be fixed with surgery and an incompetent cervix needs a stitch to strengthen it. We know that age affects our ability to have a baby, but more and more women are successfully having families in their 40s now. Hormonal irregularities can include thyroid issues, pituitary fatigue and low levels of progesterone. An endocrinologist can help with these areas.

If your progesterone levels are too low, you may not be able to carry a baby to full term. Symptoms of low progesterone include spotting and miscarriage. Low progesterone levels can also cause poor implantation in the uterus. It can be hard to diagnose progesterone deficiency during early pregnancy and so a lot of women with recurrent miscarriage are given progesterone pessaries to use as soon as they know they are pregnant and up until the end of the first trimester.

A miscarriage may start as cramping and spotting (though not all spotting is a miscarriage, and it can be normal for some women to spot during pregnancy).

Miscarriage can happen very early, and you may never know. For example, a late period that is very heavy could actually be a miscarriage.

Missed miscarriage

A missed, or silent, miscarriage is where the baby has died or not developed but has not been physically miscarried. It can be a very upsetting event because in many cases there is no sign that there was anything wrong.

In a missed miscarriage the HCG hormone can continue to be high even after the baby has died and so you may still feel pregnant, and a pregnancy test will continue to show positive. There is often no way of knowing until you have a scan.

It is devastating to go for your first scan at 12 or 13 weeks and discover that your pregnancy stopped developing days or weeks before. At a scan like this you can usually see a pregnancy sac with an embryo or foetus inside but there's no heartbeat and the pregnancy looks smaller than it should at this stage. It may also show an empty sac or no sac at all.

Your hospital team will advise you on the best route forward if this happens and you may require medication or surgery (a D and C – dilation and curettage). You may also have to return to the hospital over the course of a few weeks to make sure your HCG levels have returned to normal.

Recurrent miscarriage

Recurrent miscarriage is classified as three or more miscarriages that happen in a row.

About one in every 100 women has recurrent miscarriages. For some women, there are specific reasons for their losses but for others, those miscarriages happen by chance alone, which can be very difficult to understand. Even if you haven't been given a definite reason for your miscarriages, there is still a three out of four chance that you will go on to have a healthy birth.

Women who experience recurrent miscarriage will be linked in with a specialist service in their maternity hospital for extra care. You can also speak to your doctor about being referred to an endocrinologist to investigate if there may be a hormonal problem.

By the time women come to see me, they have usually experienced more than one miscarriage. Their obstetrician will have done the physical tests to look at the uterus and fallopian tubes and will have run chromosomal tests too.

I will take a very detailed history and listen to what happened in the months and years before the miscarriages. These histories are vital to me, they tell me so much and I work like a detective, piecing together the facts. I will know if we're looking at thyroid problems, potential pituitary fatigue or a progesterone deficiency. If I think it's that, I will give the patient progesterone pessaries from days 16 to 21 of the cycle and not just once pregnancy has occurred.

Miscarriage is one of those things that wasn't researched as well as it should have been for a long time, but thankfully, we have taken huge strides to rectify that.

Underlying hormonal problems can have an impact on all areas of your life but particularly on fertility. I would like to see women coming to see a doctor long before there is a problem getting pregnant.

I'm thankful that a lot of good people have come out and spoken about miscarriage in recent times – I love to see experiences shared. We can all learn from that.

As women, we must talk about difficult things more and normalise what happens to us and our bodies. We also need to realise that the partner of the mother who has had a miscarriage also needs support and is hurting too.

Healing

One of the first things that couples often ask is when they will be ready to try again. Physically you may be ready quite fast, but you do need to make sure that you're ready emotionally. Sometimes too, one partner is keener to try again than the other. It's very important that you discuss this and work together. It can be a stressful, emotional time and the extra stress is not going to help your hormones. Be kind to each other.

When it doesn't work

Of course, there are cases where couples have been trying for a very long time but don't have a baby. It's incredibly sad and very difficult and my heart goes out to them. They've often been on a very long road and accepting that it's not going to happen for them can be devastating.

I have seen couples who have used a donor egg and donor sperm to have their babies and couples who have completed their family with the help of a surrogate. But that is not for everyone.

Society is built around family, and that makes not having a baby when you want one a lonely place to be.

We need to value everyone equally. We used to use the village around us to raise children and hold community in high regard and I would like to see a return to that. People without children of their own are very important members of our community and should be included in the same way as everyone else.

It can take a long time to accept that you may not have children of your own and it takes time to grieve the life that you imagined, but that does not mean that life cannot be full and fun and wonderful.

CHAPTER FIVE

Perimenopause

One of the most common questions I'm asked these days is 'Am I perimenopausal?' If you have any of the symptoms listed below, the answer may be yes, and we'll address them all here.

You may not experience all of these but here are some of the symptoms you should be looking out for:

- Hot flushes
- Irregular periods
- PMS that is worse than usual
- Tiredness
- Sore or tender breasts
- Lower sex drive
- Urinary leaking when you cough or sneeze
- Needing to pee urgently

- Brain fog
- Mood swings
- Vaginal dryness or discomfort during sex
- Trouble sleeping

In the first part of perimenopause the following additional symptoms may occur or become worse:

- Heavier and longer periods
- Irritability
- Headaches and migraines
- Weight increase
- Bleeding between periods
- Bloating
- Water retention
- Increased risk of autoimmune diseases, such as Hashimoto's disease, causing an underactive thyroid

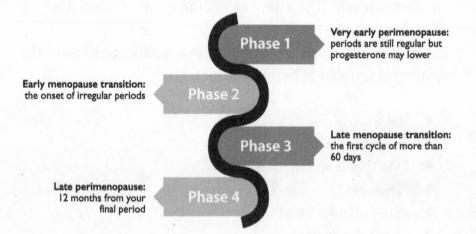

Phase 1 — Very early perimenopause: periods are still regular but progesterone may lower

Phase 2 — Early menopause transition: the onset of irregular periods

Phase 3 — Late menopause transition: the first cycle of more than 60 days

Phase 4 — Late perimenopause: 12 months from your final period

What is perimenopause?

Perimenopause is a period of transition that happens after the reproductive years but before full menopause. There are changes to the menstrual cycle where periods may become irregular; hormonal changes; and physical symptoms like hot flushes.

From as early as the age of 35, anovulatory cycles can begin. This means that ovulation does not begin every month. There are consequences as a follicle in which no egg is growing produces less or no progesterone; this causes an imbalance of the two sex hormones oestrogen and progesterone.

Symptoms of perimenopause are therefore almost always caused by a progesterone deficiency or oestrogen dominance. Perimenopause, however, does not generally occur until the age of 45 but we do occasionally see it earlier than this. Most women think that menopausal symptoms are always an oestrogen issue. However, the first hormone to take its leave is progesterone.

Common symptoms of progesterone deficiency are insomnia, anxiety and reduced resistance to stress. Decreased progesterone levels can also take away our cheerful mood and bring about low moods. For many years progesterone was only prescribed to protect the uterine lining. This is certainly one therapeutic effect of progesterone but it has many other positive effects on the mind and nervous system.

Perimenopause will usually last between three and five years. At this time our egg reserves become depleted in the ovary. As that happens the FSH levels rise in the pituitary gland. If women are overdoing it, which they usually are, they have a tired pituitary gland to begin with so there is already a hormonal imbalance.

This hormonal imbalance impacts the nerve–muscle junction and can cause muscle pain, IBS, restless sleep and restless legs, sweating and palpitations. Insomnia caused by all of these symptoms then exacerbates the pituitary fatigue further and the symptoms get worse.

One of the symptoms that patients find most difficult to deal with is brain fog. Although not a clinical diagnosis, brain fog is usually defined by forgetfulness, distractedness, sluggishness and a feeling of being overwhelmed. Patients worry that they are getting early dementia, which of course they are not. What is happening is that they are exhausted because of lack of sleep and anxiety, and the brain messaging and synapses slow down. Once you correct the hormonal imbalance and make patients realise that they must pace themselves and make lifestyle changes to recharge their hormone control centre, the brain fog usually lifts.

After years of no one even acknowledging the time before menopause, perimenopause is having a moment. There are now articles, books and TV programmes about it, and I am thrilled.

It has been my mission for years to educate women and doctors about perimenopause and menopause. I've been talking about it at events, conferences, on the radio, on TV and in print. I have always said that the more we know, the better armed we are to deal with what's going on.

Aisling Grimley, who created the website *My Second Spring*, telling her own story of early menopause, invited me to give a lecture on menopause in the Merrion Hotel in Dublin and it was there that I met Lorraine Keane. From then, our shared journey of educating women was written in the stars.

Melanie Morris, who had organised the Network for Women with *Image*, asked me to give a lecture to 300 women in Dublin's Marker Hotel in 2014. Those women had a huge appetite for knowledge about their hormonal health and from there the seed was sown.

I knew that this was the correct journey to go on. We had to educate the public and change the narrative to create change and give rise to the wonderful awareness of perimenopause and menopause that we have today.

With the help of Lorraine Keane, I have travelled the country over the past eight years because I wanted to change the narrative and taboo about menopause. I had heard too much of the terrible suffering that women endured, but the only way to change things was by getting out and educating the public that menopause is nothing to be ashamed of and that it is a natural phenomenon.

The interest in these public lectures was phenomenal and drove me to educate more. I did hormone health podcasts with Lorraine and was a contributor to *Let's Talk Hormone Health*. These podcasts are free to download from my website.

Going on *Liveline* with Joe Duffy on RTÉ Radio 1 was a major game changer as it has such a broad reach. It opened a real can of worms. Women came on with dreadful stories of how they had suffered severely with no help. They had not been listened to. They described how they were going from pillar to post complaining of severe muscle pain, brain fog, lack of sleep, palpitations, sensitive skin, first-time allergies and weight gain and had been treated like hypochondriacs.

When I put it all together and demonstrated the hormonal link that this was part of the hormonal imbalance that occurs in perimenopause and menopause, they sighed with relief, happy to know that they weren't losing it.

Even just a decade ago, you would have thought that women went from 15 to 55 in the height of fertility with not a bother on them. The years before menopause were completely discounted. If you were tired, emotional, stressed or confused about what was happening to your body, you were dismissed or told you were depressed.

Not only did people not realise what perimenopause is, but they also didn't realise how big it is and how much of an impact it has on women's lives. We had been taught that menopause was when our periods stopped, and that is true, but we were never taught about the years before that when everything starts to change. It can be as important for many women as menopause itself.

Women should have been told that hormonal changes do not start with menopause when their periods stop but much earlier. Then they would understand that overdoing it at work and as a mother is putting pressure on their hormonal systems, as their FSH levels are rising and in flux while the eggs in their ovaries are depleting.

You would understand that having a glass of wine in the evening was amplifying your oestrogen dominance at this time and that all the extra oestrogen and cortisol in the blood due to stress was putting too much pressure on your hormonal system.

CASE HISTORY: CIARA

Ciara was 37 years old and came to me with disrupted sleep, night sweats, irregular periods, severe fatigue and (for the first time in her life) severe anxiety. She also had a low libido and her relationship with her partner was suffering,

I suspected that she might have been experiencing premature menopause. The laboratory confirmed this, as her progesterone level was barely detectable and her oestrogen levels were also very low.

I advised her on lifestyle change and diet but I also prescribed HRT. She was already on MenoMin, which is a supplement for perimenopause and menopause with vitamin D, omega 3, biotin, vitamins B6 and B12 and natural phytoestrogens.

Her condition stabilised from week to week, and she did very well. Her sleep and concentration improved immeasurably. She also practised meditation and yoga, which she found very beneficial.

Symptoms of perimenopause

It is important that you know the symptoms of perimenopause so that you can understand the changes your body is going through and avoid any unnecessary alarm. Women often fear the worst when they get new symptoms and, instead of thinking about perimenopause, they panic.

You might see physical symptoms like brittle or thinning hair, dull-looking skin, bladder leakages or vaginal dryness or you might experience emotional changes like low mood, low sexual desire and libido, a change in sleeping patterns or brain fog.

Not a lot of people speak about how perimenopause can affect your hair and skin, but it is an important symptom to acknowledge. It doesn't happen overnight, but it can be something that you suddenly notice. You might look in the mirror and think you look old and that can have a huge emotional impact. Perimenopause is very like a second puberty. There are huge emotional and physical changes and that can be an awful lot to deal with.

But knowledge is power. If you can recognise the symptoms of perimenopause and menopause, you can self-advocate. Some doctors might dismiss tiredness or brain fog, but if you know it's not normal for you and you think it could be your hormones, you will be able to push for tests or medication. We women know ourselves better than anyone else and that is a very powerful tool. Remember we are amazing nurturers to others and we can be the same to ourselves.

Information and knowledge are key to reclaiming our power and to understanding our hormonal selves at this time in our lives. We are now learning that there is no shame in being at the mercy of hormones as we now know how powerful they are and that they control both men and women. We need to get people to question their hormones more.

We need doctors to consider hormones more when they are treating women above 35 and sometimes even younger, as I occasionally see perimenopause in women in their 20s. It all goes back to our training. Listen to the patient. Check her menstrual history. Make sure to take a comprehensive history and do not dismiss her hormones. With so many cases that I encounter in my daily practice hormones must be factored in as a cause within the treatment strategy.

When does perimenopause start?

Perimenopause normally begins from the age of 45 onwards but in some women can happen much earlier. A lot of what happens at this time is genetic and if your mother had an early menopause, then that follows on to the next generation too. That's another good reason to speak up about women's health. Your mum can shed so much light on your family history and help you prepare for what's to come.

The other main factor that can influence when you might start perimenopause is if you smoke. Smokers reach menopause about two years earlier than other women.

For a long time, this period of life was seen as the end of something, but I like to view it as the start of something new. Change is good, it is exciting, and this is a new chapter in our lives, the second half of our lives. It should be celebrated! The way you frame something in your mind has a lot to do with how you experience it. If you're already dreading perimenopause and treat it as something sad or bad, it will be harder to get through your symptoms. Positivity goes a long way in helping you deal with a hard time.

It's a time in our lives when we could do with a bit of understanding and kindness, which is why I'd like to see men educated on the subject. I'd also like it talked about more in a work setting so that people can understand what their female colleagues are going through.

Things like hot flushes can be embarrassing at work but would be less so if it was just seen as a normal health issue. So little is understood by people about what happens to a woman during menopause that we're often expected to simply carry on through our symptoms, but that can be really hard to do.

There are the hot flushes but there's also exhaustion, brain fog and sometimes pain and that can make work difficult. Women can feel embarrassed, upset and worried about their careers. If open conversations were to happen around menopause, so many women would feel more supported by their employers. I'm so happy to see some large companies offer menopause leave now, but I believe that real progress can only happen when we normalise perimenopause and menopause.

Ways to help

It will come as absolutely no surprise to you by now that I'm going to talk to you about rest. The right amount of good-quality rest is vital at this stage in your life as FSH levels are rising in the pituitary gland, and the hormone control centre copes better when it is recharged. It also avoids other hormones, such as adrenaline, being released in excess and upsetting the hormone balance when you are overtired.

When a woman comes to see me with concerns about perimenopause or menopause the first thing I speak to them about is rest. How are they sleeping? Are they being supported at work and at home? Can they take it a bit easier? It's often a hard time for slowing down. Women in their late 40s might have a young family that keeps them very active or elderly parents that they help to look after, but the importance of rest cannot be underestimated.

Remember how much you slept as a teenager? Or how much our teens sleep now? They need that to help their bodies and brains cope with all the hormonal changes that are happening – and you need it too.

If you're symptomatic and struggling, there are a couple of options. We've all heard of HRT, which is great and very necessary for some women. If you have vaginal dryness, which is a very common symptom and can affect your sex life, oestrogen pessaries can be used.

Supplements can help during perimenopause. Vitamins B6 and B12 help nervous function; vitamin D is essential for bone growth, and you need this because as oestrogen levels drop you lose bone mass. Omega 3 is important for heart function. Isoflavones are a natural oestrogen; they are classified as phytoestrogens or plant-derived compounds with oestrogenic activity.

There are good supplements on the market that have all of these in them. When it comes to supplements it's a good idea to speak to your doctor about them. Some can interfere with medication and some should be taken in specific dose amounts so it's wise to have a conversation with your doctor before you start taking any of them.

I find that many women do quite well with rest, a supplement and taking something for restless legs, but other women have more severe symptoms and need the help of HRT.

It's also important to have a healthy diet so that you get adequate minerals and vitamins and to keep sugar in your diet low at this time. Magnesium is also a good supplement to take at this time as it helps with muscle relaxation and thus sleep. I will talk about this more later in the book.

Common body changes during perimenopause

Every woman is different and many women say that they have no physical symptoms during perimenopause other than irregular periods. But for lots of women there are notable changes and navigating their way through those can be difficult. Things like hot flushes, night sweating and the much-dreaded vaginal dryness can be shocking to experience at first.

There are gradients to these symptoms too. They can be mild for some and more difficult to manage for others. The most important thing to remember is that these are natural, normal changes and you are not the only woman to be experiencing them.

Hot flushes

These are what you hear about the most when you start to discuss perimenopause and menopause with your family and friends. They occur due to oestrogen deficiency.

They don't happen for everyone but for the women who do experience them, they're uncomfortable, unpleasant, and sometimes embarrassing. They can happen at any time of the day, often without warning and at inconvenient times.

This besets 90% of us. A hot flush starts with a sudden wave of heat and is usually accompanied by sweating, going red and a rapid heartbeat. Some women also feel a tingling in their fingers. They usually last between one and five minutes, which doesn't sound like long but it's long enough when you're in the middle of one. They can happen a couple of times a day right up to 20 times a day. They usually do not cause any body odour.

They are a reaction to the hormonal decline going on in your body – think of it as if the thermostat in your brain has broken and has forgotten how to work properly.

Common triggers can include alcohol, caffeine, spicy foods, stress, tight clothes, smoking (or being in a smoky environment) and being in a hot room.

You might also experience them at night in bed which can interfere with your rest. These are called night sweats. As warmth is followed by cold a lot of women wake up at night shivering as they are drenched in sweat and feel cold. I have often come across patients who have had to change nightwear several times in the night. Perimenopausal women are often painted as irritable, but wouldn't you be irritable if you were living with hot flushes and night sweats and getting little sleep?

How to help relieve hot flushes

- Keep iced water on hand and sip it at the start of a hot flush.
- Dress in layers, even if it's cold outside. Hot flushes aren't weather-dependent so the last thing you want to do is be caught wearing a wool jumper you can't take off.
- If you're getting them at night, wear cotton nightclothes and make sure your sheets are cotton. Breathable fabrics are much better at keeping us cool.
- Bring a cool pack to bed with you to help lower your temperature and get you back to sleep.

Lifestyle changes to help to reduce the longevity of hot flushes

- Eat a well-balanced diet with controlled portion sizes and stay away from spicy or other trigger foods.
- Soy contains phytoestrogens which act like oestrogen in the body. Soy is particularly high in isoflavones, which bind to oestrogen receptors. This can help reduce hot flushes. Some good dietary sources of soy include soy milk, tofu and edamame beans.
- Get regular exercise. It's always used as the answer to everything, but it genuinely does help.
- Try to control your stress. Yoga, meditation and time to decompress all help to lessen the symptoms.

Oestrogen deficiency can trigger other symptoms aside from hot flushes including:

- Irritability
- Restlessness
- Cardiovascular disease
- Osteoporosis
- Increase in facial hair
- Sinking breast tissue
- Insomnia
- Forgetfulness
- Urge to urinate
- Urinary tract infections
- Dry skin and mucous membranes
- Dry eyes
- Thinning skin
- Hair loss
- Change in vaginal flora
- Decreased blood circulation to the vagina
- Vaginal infections
- Stress incontinence

Vaginal atrophy

The drop in oestrogen levels we experience in perimenopause and menopause can lead to vaginal atrophy. It sounds terrifying, as you might understand 'atrophy' to mean wasting away and so fear the worst, but it's basically the thinning and drying of the tissues of the vagina.

If left untreated, it can cause a feeling of vaginal tightness, burning or pain during sex, urinary tract infections and frequent urination. Though the term is still used, there is a newer term for the condition that you may start to hear more often: genito-urinary syndrome of menopause (GSM).

You can use over-the-counter lubricants to help with the dryness and to relieve pain during sex, while women with more severe symptoms of the condition may need to be prescribed localised oestrogen products.

Urinary and bladder issues

Because oestrogen has a role in keeping our pelvic floor healthy, some women also experience problems with incontinence and increased numbers of urinary tract infections (UTIs). I'll explain more about this in the chapter on menopause.

Fibroids

It is estimated that between 70% and 80% of all women will develop fibroids by the time they're 50 and, because many women don't have any symptoms, that number may actually be higher. They can be very small or big enough to change the shape of your uterus and are benign tumours that very rarely develop into cancer. Lots of women are surprised to find they have fibroids when they're being examined for something else.

So what is the link between perimenopause and fibroids? Well, simply put, perimenopause makes them worse. If you have a fibroid, the onset of perimenopause can make them grow significantly because of a surplus of oestrogen in the years before menopause. In these years, your menstrual cycle is dominated by oestrogen and so they have the perfect place to grow. Depending on where they are, they can cause prolonged, heavy periods, and pain and/or pressure on your lower back and abdomen. They can also cause bleeding between periods. If that is happening, you must speak to your doctor so that they can rule out other causes.

Historically the treatment for fibroids was a hysterectomy, which we all know is an incredibly invasive major surgery and so a lot of women waited to have anything done. There are alternative treatments now that stop menstruation and help the fibroid tissue to shrink, and focused ultrasounds that can treat smaller ones. You can now have an embolisation, which is a minimally invasive treatment that halts the blood flow to targeted areas and blocks the blood vessels. You can have your fibroids surgically removed. The Mirena coil (which releases progesterone slowly over five years) will shrink them (in most cases).

All of these procedures are preferable to a hysterectomy.

What I hope would become the norm in the future, though, is controlling overly heavy periods from the very beginning. If we can do that, we can stop FSH over-pumping and reduce the chance of fibroids forming in the first place.

The language of perimenopause and menopause

We know that words matter and for a long time menopause has been spoken about as if it's a very funny joke. Saying things like 'She's mad' or 'She's going through "the change"' have been used as ways to mock women at this time of their lives.

Even the word hysterectomy has a part to play in this. The word hysteria comes from the Greek root *hystera*, which means uterus. It was believed that hysteria was caused by a defect in the uterus and that only women could become hysterical. In the late 1800s, doctors cured the hysteria of women by removing what they believed to be the cause, the uterus, and so the word hysterectomy came to be.

A lot of younger physicians are fighting to have the procedure renamed because of its sexist origins and would prefer it to now be called a uterectomy. Interestingly, and a little depressingly, hysterectomy is only used when talking about the procedure for women; in female animals, it's already called a uterectomy.

Flooding

Something that happens a lot that you may not have heard of at all is flooding. About a quarter of all perimenopausal women will experience heavy bleeding, which is also known as hypermenorrhoea, menorrhagia or flooding. For some women, their periods are so heavy during perimenopause that even the biggest pads can't contain them.

It happens because, as your body tries to make your ovaries release an egg, your oestrogen levels rise, causing your uterine lining to thicken, but because women who aren't ovulating any more don't always produce enough progesterone to balance out the oestrogen, you get an unusually thick lining which sheds differently from how it used to. You might have very large clots or sudden gushes of blood that are too much for your sanitary protection to contain.

This can cause you to become anaemic, feel faint and have a lower blood volume. Taking an NSAID (non-steroidal anti-inflammatory) every four to six hours during a very heavy period can reduce blood loss, or your doctor might prescribe you mefenamic acid (you might know it as Ponstan).

Hormonal coils like Mirena, Kyleena or Jaydess can help and so too can the combined oral contraceptive pill. Progesterone-only pills or implants can also be effective, as can some forms of HRT.

We've come a long way in discussing perimenopausal symptoms, but we could go further. I'd hazard a guess that a lot of women have not heard of flooding. Menstrual blood is one of the great taboos and that is something we need to change.

Signs that you may be experiencing flooding

- You're changing your sanitary wear more frequently or are having to double up on protection.
- Your period is lasting more than seven days.
- You're passing large clots.
- Your periods are more painful than before.
- You have blood flooding through your sanitary protection and onto your clothes during the day.
- Your bedclothes are soaked with blood at night.

Migraine

For lots of women who have experienced some form of hormone-related headaches during their life, perimenopause can trigger an increase in migraines. The rise and fall in oestrogen and progesterone levels can mean that migraine sufferers see a worsening of their headaches or an increase in their frequency. Iron deficiency from dysfunctional bleeding or heavy periods can also cause an increase in migraines.

Your GP will have a lot of treatments for migraine, but natural methods include taking magnesium and vitamin B12. It's good to check if your B12 levels are normal because this vitamin normalises the production of serotonin and improves the function of an enzyme which has been linked to migraines. HRT can also improve migraines for some women, though it can worsen them in others.

Migraines are hormonal and can happen in mid-cycle or ovulation, but they happen any time there's a hormonal imbalance. It's the most common headache that you would get in perimenopause and menopause.

Lack of sleep

Progesterone calms the nerves and affects many parts of the body. Approximately half of all menopausal women experience some form of insomnia and progesterone treatment can be very beneficial for this.

The calming and anxiety-relieving effect is transmitted through allopregnanolone, the neurosteroid metabolite of progesterone. This nerve agent is claimed to have an anti-depressant effect and be effective against other mental disorders too.

Peripheral circulatory problems can be a cause of poor sleep for women going through perimenopause and menopause, and progesterone also helps with circulation to alleviate such problems.

Progesterone helps you fall asleep faster and above all helps you sleep deeply during the first half of the night. Canadian researchers found that eight hours of sleep promotes optimal weight regulation. Those who had been getting too little sleep over several years had an almost 30% risk of gaining 5kg over a six-year period. Leptin levels drop if you suffer sleep deprivation. In addition, too much appetite-stimulating ghrelin is being formed.

Sleep tips

- The bedroom should be cool, dark and quiet.
- Ban all electrical devices before falling asleep.
- Your cortisol level is highest one or two hours after waking up and allows you to launch into the day. Cortisol is also released during sporting activity, so try not to do any vigorous exercise after 7 p.m. An exercise like gentle yoga is more calming.
- Avoid caffeine before bedtime, as it lowers melatonin levels and therefore makes falling asleep more difficult.
- Warm milk with honey before bedtime is good as milk contains melatonin and tryptophan (which also increases melatonin).
- Consuming a rich diet or a late meal in the evening also affects the quality of our sleep. In particular, highly processed sugar and carbohydrates can lead to insulin release and subsequent hypoglycaemia and thus can disrupt your sleep.
- Try to spend as much time as you can outdoors during the day as it promotes Vitamin D production and also suppresses melatonin and makes you more alert.
- Try to go to sleep by 11 p.m. and definitely before midnight.

Perimenopausal mood disorders

Mood disorders, including depression, are more common during the perimenopausal years than during the pre- or postmenopausal years. The risk for new-onset depression is approximately 30%, and for women with a prior history of depression, the risk is 60%. Rates then decrease in the post-menopause years.

Although the risk of mood disorders is high, screening rates for depression tend to be low. In a survey of 500 practising obstetrician gynaecologists (with a 42% response rate, 209 of 500), most physicians routinely screened perimenopausal women for depression, but over one-third of the respondents (34%, 71 of 209) did not. In addition, while the majority of respondents (86%, 178 of 209) believed that they could recognise depression in perimenopausal women, only approximately one-half (56%, 117 of 209) felt confident in their ability to manage these patients. These observations highlight the need for improved education of physicians about the importance of routine screening for and management of mood disorders during the menopausal transition.

How you deal with these episodes of depression hormone imbalance depends on how severe they are. If the depression is mild and they don't have any hot flushes, many women cope by using mindfulness practices like yoga, exercise and meditation. If the depression is more serious and there are also other symptoms like hot flushes or sleeplessness, HRT may be the appropriate intervention.

I always try to see the patient as a whole and treat the bigger picture. If I think a woman in my clinic is depressed but her hot flushes are not severe, I try to treat the other symptoms first. Does she have restless legs that are keeping her awake at night and exacerbating her tiredness and therefore her hormonal imbalance?

It's important to look at every element. Finding the root cause is my first step, and I like to treat that rather than the symptom. That way we get better results and find out what's really going on.

Reactive depression is a hormonal imbalance

Depression is overdiagnosed in women. If we have very heavy periods, it causes a hormonal imbalance, which affects our hormonal circadian rhythm and results in fatigue. This does not mean we are depressed.

I vividly recall the late Professor Anthony Clare teaching us the difference between endogenous and reactive depression. If you are fed up with being tired and have total insight into your condition, it is highly likely that you have a hormonal imbalance causing fatigue, not depression.

I remember when I gave birth to my twin boys prematurely. It was very traumatic because I had to have an emergency caesarean and one of my boys was put on a ventilator for three weeks as he had respiratory distress syndrome. It was touch and go and I was woken up at 3 a.m. by the consultant paediatrician on call to say they had been in contact with Great Ormond Street Children's Hospital in London; his oxygen saturations were dropping and the only chance he had was to be put on an oscillator to help his lungs to work. The complication of that was that he was at risk of a bleed into the brain due to a potential rise of intracranial pressure. I was terrified and stressed but I had to give my consent as it was the only chance my little boy had. I prayed so hard that he would be all right.

I was already exhausted after the emergency section and was now having to deal with this. I got severe maternity blues because my hormone control centre was exhausted. Once I was given the chance to rest, I was fine.

I believe post-natal depression is not depression but hormonal imbalance. Long sleep deprivation caused by pregnancy, labour and motherhood leads to hormonal imbalance causing severe fatigue and insomnia due to peripheral nerve pain, and all this exacerbates the fatigue more. It's not just my opinion, though; there have been studies done on the link between post-natal depression and hormonal imbalance, including one called *The Role of Reproductive Hormones in Postpartum Depression* published by Cambridge University Press in 2014.

After having a long labour, which most women do, preceded by poor sleeping in the months before having the baby, women are tired. Maternity hospitals are wonderful places with fantastic teams working in them but new mothers do not get the support that they need. Our maternity hospitals need to be better resourced to allow women to get the rest they need after a long labour and delivery.

Currently, in Ireland, new mothers who have had an uncomplicated vaginal birth are discharged from hospital within 24 hours and those who have had a caesarean section stay in hospital between three and five days. In the public system, new mothers have a six-week check-up at their GP surgery. There are also visits from the public health nurse.

In the past, maternity hospitals had a nursery where babies were looked after so that new mothers could get some much-needed rest. Women don't get that now and often leave hospital totally exhausted after labour or surgery and go home to night feeds and months of disturbed sleep. The nurses and staff in all our maternity hospitals are excellent and give great quality care but they need more help. We need more audits and to listen to both sides.

Also, as women, we have seen our mothers do most of the work getting up at night and rearing the children. Thankfully, times are changing and now fathers have become more involved. I always recommend that a mother gets the first few nights to sleep uninterrupted to charge her batteries and then for the couple to take turns doing the feeds every second night so that neither of them gets burnout.

I am a big advocate of breastfeeding but it does mean that your nights are interrupted, so make sure you get plenty of lie-ins and that you have a supportive partner who realises that you must recharge properly. Your new baby is most definitely a full-time job!

CASE HISTORY: EIMEAR

Eimear came to see me with an awful story. Her last child was 5.7kg (12lb 10oz), a very large baby, and when she was having him the midwife told her to have one last big push. That push resulted in a massive tear, right back to the anus, and she had had a terrible time ever since.

She had severe incontinence, a huge problem with intercourse because the stitching after the tear was too tight, and she had a uterine prolapse. As a result of the prolapse, she had a hysterectomy and the surgeon also took out her ovaries. She wasn't put on HRT afterwards and went into sudden menopause, which is not at all physiological.

I saw her 12 years later with very severe symptoms of menopause. She had osteoporosis and had developed Type 2 diabetes five years previously because her metabolism crashed after sudden surgical menopause, and she put on a lot of weight.

All of this suffering shouldn't have happened to this woman. It stemmed from the size of her baby. They would have known the size of the baby at 37 weeks and she should never have been put through that. She should have been offered a caesarian section and not have been made to deliver a baby of that size vaginally. No woman would be able to deliver a child of that size without doing themselves some damage. Introducing her to a physiotherapist during her pregnancy would have helped her improve her pelvic muscles and helped in this decision process. As a result of the long labour, her baby also had to be admitted to the neonatal intensive care unit for a week, which was very distressing.

We have to stop the guilt around having a caesarean; if you need one you need one and that should be the end of it. Of course, having our baby naturally and vaginally is what most of us desire but in some cases, it is not possible.

We need to empower women around maternal healthcare and allow them to feel confident enough to ask how they're going to deliver very large babies.

Eimear is on HRT now, seeing a pelvic floor physio and we're working on her diabetes and other symptoms, but she may need a repair surgery for her prolapse in the future.

CASE HISTORY: ELEANOR

Eleanor was 46 when she came to me with severe fatigue and anxiety.

Extensive blood tests including FSH, LH and thyroid function did not reveal any abnormality. However, she did have low progesterone. She was having regular periods but there were some cycles without ovulation which were causing progesterone deficiency. She did very well on progesterone therapy and changes to her lifestyle.

Contraception in perimenopause

A lot of women in their 40s ask me about contraception and whether it's okay to still be on the pill or use a coil. It is okay and women who are still having regular sex and don't want to become pregnant must remember that they're still fertile. It's important to continue to remember that hormonal contraception does not protect against STIs, and if you have new or different partners you should be using barrier methods (condoms).

As you know by now, I would prefer to see men who have completed their families have a vasectomy so that their partners can stop taking hormonal contraception. Women still need some form of contraception for a year after their last period as protection from pregnancy and it would be preferable for men to take charge of that. Women have borne the burden of contraception for so long and it bothers me so much that men still won't step up and have a simple procedure that allows their partners to stop having to worry.

That being said, it is still fine to use hormonal contraception into your 40s. My preference would be the Mirena coil or the progesterone-only pill for women of this age.

Testosterone

There has been much discussion about testosterone therapy lately and its use for the treatment of menopausal women. It can be used for the low libido that is often a symptom of perimenopause and menopause.

It can be given once a day in a pea-sized amount and you don't get the side effects of acne or excess hair at that level. Many women have experienced great success with it. It is currently not licensed for use in that way in Ireland and so is something to discuss with your doctor.

We need a lot more research in this area as sexual desire and health are a part of normal society and when libido lowers in women due to hormonal imbalance we need to have answers to help them. We also need to do the same for men.

CASE HISTORY: NIAMH

Niamh was 44 and had two young children. She came to see me complaining of disturbed sleep, night sweats, a lack of motivation, loss of libido, brain fog and anxiety.

Her relationship with her husband had been affected because she had no interest in sex any more. She was very irritable and short-tempered with her kids, which was upsetting her. Her professional life was also affected by her exhaustion and irritability.

I thought she was in perimenopause and the laboratory tests I ran confirmed my suspicion. I treated her with HRT, vitamin D and magnesium. She returned to her old self and we were both delighted with the results.

Forty-four may seem young to be perimenopausal but it can happen and it's one of the reasons I ask you to keep in tune with your body. Recognising small changes can go a long way to getting the help you might need.

CHAPTER SIX

Menopause

Konenki

The Japanese word for menopause is *konenki* but it doesn't mean menopause as we know it. Instead of being the pause or end of something, *konenki* is a time for newness. *Ko* means renewal or regeneration. *Nen* is years and *Ki* is a season or an energy. As a word, it is used less to describe the end of menstruation and more generally about a time of transition. It is thought that having a more positive word for the experience frames it totally differently in one's culture and that cultural significance can change everything.

At this point in my career, a lot of my public work is focused on menopause and I'm very passionate about it. It will come as no surprise to you that I am a fan of education on menopause as I have heard too many stories of women who have suffered. For a long time, there has been a stigma around what is a natural, biological process that every woman you know has experienced or will experience. It is my great passion to make sure that both my medical colleagues and women are armed with as much information about what happens at this crucial time as possible. Thankfully, a lot has improved in this area since I started touring the country eight years ago with Lorraine Keane.

It can be a difficult time with symptoms that are often tricky to live with but it is also a time of opportunity, change and growth.

In Asia, they call menopause the Second Spring, which I love. It astounds me how long it took us to see it as a natural phenomenon and we can learn a lot about how framing it more positively can change the experience for many women. Menopause is part of the natural evolutionary process, so why did it take us so long to be empowered and educated about it?

Menopause is nothing new; it is as old as the human race. It's time to reclaim this chapter in our lives as something positive and an experience to be celebrated.

So, what is menopause?

Menopause is the end of your menstrual cycle. It is diagnosed when you have gone a full year without a period. The average age for menopause is 51 but it can happen at any time from your mid-40s. Before the conversation around perimenopause grew, many people assumed that menopause just lasted a long time. We are more educated about what happens now but there is still a lot of work to do.

The portrayal of menopausal women on television, in cinema and in the media has traditionally been one of a haggard, out-of-date, grey-haired, angry woman, and that must change. Some of the happiest, most vibrant women I know are menopausal!

If you are lucky enough to not have many symptoms in perimenopause, you might not even realise you are going through it. Because cycles become irregular as you age you might have a period and assume there will be another in a few months; few of us will note the exact day we had our final period at the time. It's only in hindsight when none show up that we might realise, that's it, we're done.

To find out you are in menopause our doctor will take a good history and also check your hormones via a blood test. They will check if your periods have stopped and if you have any other symptoms.

One of the reasons I started out speaking to doctors about menopause is that a lot of medical professionals haven't had specific menopausal training. They either may not know all the symptoms or think that they're easy to live with. There also was not enough emphasis and research on women's health. That attitude has caused suffering for many women and thankfully GPs offer better care around menopause now.

The stages and symptoms

We have already spoken about symptoms in the chapter on perimenopause but there is more to menopausal symptoms than the hot flushes that are widely talked about.

Oestrogen is a very powerful hormone and as it declines in our perimenopausal years it can set off a whole host of symptoms. In menopause, we must look after our mind, our brain, our bones, our muscles and joints, our vagina, our bladder, our heart, our weight, our skin, our hair and our rest.

That sounds like a long list of things that we must pay attention to, doesn't it? But we've been minding those things all our lives and we just have to learn how to mind them a little differently now.

As a child, you paid little or no heed to any of those. As you entered puberty and things changed you learned how to manage all of them differently; you just forget what that was like because it feels so long ago. That was a time of great excitement as you became a woman, and this stage of life should be no different. Instead of viewing it with dread, we should be excited to enter this next phase.

You might need some lifestyle changes, you might need some medication or you might need a holiday with the girls and to let your hair down! So much of life is about attitude and we must change ours when it comes to menopause.

Some women find it useful to note down their symptoms and keep a diary of how they are feeling. It can be a very useful tool, especially if you need to speak to a doctor about what's going on. It can be easy to forget everything you'd like to say when you get into a clinic for an appointment and a chart of symptoms can be a great way to run through everything.

As you know, I'm passionate about taking a good history from a patient and if a woman comes to me with a symptom diary I am delighted.

Menopause

You can find a lot of lists online that you can print off to rate your symptoms. Here is mine:

0 = none   1 = mild   2 = medium   3 = severe

Symptoms	0	1	2	3
Hot flushes				
Night sweats				
Fatigue				
Brain fog*				
Insomnia				
Restless legs				
Nerve pain**				
Loss of libido				
Anxiety				
Lack of interest				
Feeling unusually emotional				
Headaches				
Palpitations				
Vaginal dryness				
Vaginal pain				
Sadness				

* Brain fog can include those times when it's hard to concentrate or you're talking and suddenly find yourself searching for a word.

** Peripheral nerve pain is often felt in the fingers and feet but can also be experienced as tingling in the limbs, coldness and numbness.

Global menopause study

The beauty company Avon conducted a large survey about perimenopause and menopause in 2020. The study, called *Menopause TLI. Too Little Information: The global conversation deficit* found that more than two-fifths (44%) of women around the world were unaware of perimenopause and menopause right up until they started having symptoms themselves.

A third of women said that they were getting most of their information online ahead of gynaecologists, endocrinologists, GPs and friends.

Perimenopause came as a particular shock with almost half of those surveyed (46%) saying they did not expect it when it started; and 44% of the women felt anxious during perimenopause.

There was an overall lack of understanding of menopause and its stages. More than one-third (36%) of the women surveyed didn't understand the two phases, perimenopause and menopause, even while in the midst of one of the phases themselves, and 46% did not feel prepared for menopause.

The study showed that around the world menopause is still a subject women are reluctant to discuss and would rather turn to the internet than speak to medical professionals, friends or family.

Although it is widely known that perimenopause and menopause often follow maternal patterns, only 6% of the survey respondents said that they would discuss it with their mother.

Almost a quarter of the women said that they would feel uncomfortable speaking to their partner about menopause, and, shockingly, 22% of them said that they even felt uncomfortable discussing it with friends.

It also found that twice as many women in the UK were more likely to get their information from the internet (53%) than from a doctor (24%).

Menopausal symptoms

Let's talk about time. Usually, you're perimenopausal for between three and five years before you hit menopause. A lot of women believe that because your periods stop when you arrive at menopause, that's it, you're out of the woods, but you can still carry on having menopausal symptoms for five years after the cessation of your periods.

That means some women can have varying degrees of symptoms for 10 years. That is a long time in your life, which is why the more you know and understand early on, the faster you can get help if you need it and regain control of your body and life.

We've already discussed hot flushes, night sweats and low mood in relation to perimenopause so let's now talk about some of the other big symptoms you may get in your menopausal years.

Brain fog

This is a big one and can be upsetting for many women. I've often had patients come to see me in a panic talking about early-onset dementia. Intelligent, successful, eloquent women who now find themselves struggling to find a simple word, remember a name or having to read the same page over and over again arrive at my clinic feeling devastated. It can lead to embarrassing situations at work and to social anxiety and it is difficult to understand and experience.

The good news is that it's not dementia, but it is a real symptom of menopause and it's down to your hormones. Several hormones work in unison to keep your mind clear. When even one of them is out of balance it creates a knock-on effect.

Cortisol, serotonin and dopamine all play a part in keeping your brain ticking over and it's easy for them to become disrupted. Oestrogen also plays a part in brain activity and enhances the neurotransmitters that improve memory and learning. When your oestrogen levels drop in menopause your brain is affected alongside everything else.

On top of all of this, your brain needs good-quality rest to process and repair each night. When you're not getting that rest because of night sweats, restless legs or peripheral nerve pain, everything slows down, including brain synapses.

If brain fog is an issue, you should first look at your rest and see what can be improved there. If you can't sleep because of those menopausal symptoms, speak to your doctor about treatments that can help you. Magnesium is a lovely supplement to take at night that helps to relax your muscles. When calcium binds to proteins such as troponin C and myosin, this process changes the shape of these proteins, generating a contraction. Magnesium competes with calcium for these same binding spots to help relax your muscles

If you are stressed or anxious, try to calm yourself before sleep. Take a few hours in the evening to completely relax, try meditation and yoga and see if it helps to ease the fog.

Remember too that the brain is a muscle as well as an organ, and one that you cannot just ignore as you come into your second spring. Word and number games, reading and brain training all make a big difference in keeping your brain functioning well, so ignore it at your peril!

Breast changes

If you have had children, you'll have some experience with your breasts' ability to change completely. These changes continue as you hit menopause.

Loss of breast fullness is common at this time and is a result of how falling oestrogen levels change the milk system in our breasts. They may start to droop, lose their round shape and you might find lumps in them. This is usually nothing to worry about, but lumps can be frightening and you should see your doctor if you're worried.

Skin and hair

Skin and hair changes might sound like very superficial symptoms to be worried about when there is so much going on in your body and mind but they're very important in how you feel, which makes them very important to talk about.

I mentioned these changes in the perimenopause chapter but let's look at them in more detail. Because they seem trivial women are afraid to bring them up when discussing symptoms, but they shouldn't be. If you're already struggling with the changes in your body, seeing your hair and skin look different or older can be incredibly upsetting.

Our skin cells contain oestrogen receptors which control

things like sebum (which keeps skin lubricated), hyaluronic acid (which grabs onto the moisture in our skin and helps reduce the appearance of fine lines), ceramides (which helps protect your skin) and collagen (which gives your skin fullness and strength).

When those oestrogen levels drop, all these functions are impacted. What you can be left with is dull, dry skin that is starting to droop and looks more wrinkled than before. Some women also see a return to the acne they may have had in puberty because the change in sebum production can lead to blocked follicles and spots.

So what can you do? You'll probably have seen a lot of skincare products that contain hyaluronic acid and ceramides, and for good reason. Both are a great addition to your skincare routine and help return moisture and plumpness to the skin and add a protective barrier. Remember to apply your hyaluronic acid product to damp skin so that it can grab that moisture inwards. Also, remember to wear a high-factor, broad-spectrum sun cream every day; menopausal skin contains less melanin, which protects us from sun damage, so it is more vulnerable to UV rays.

Some brands have brought out specific ranges for menopausal skin and it's a wonderful thing to see. While you don't necessarily need to pay big money for skincare or buy those specific ranges, the very fact that big brands see the market for them means that menopause is becoming talked about and normalised.

It's not just the skin on your face that changes, the skin on some women's bodies becomes very itchy and dry too and can be very uncomfortable. This is called pruritus. You can become much more sensitive to fragranced products, creams and detergents, so choosing unscented options for sensitive skin can help. If the itching is interfering with your sleep, it's time to see your doctor, who can talk through medicated options with you.

During the menopause and perimenopause years, some women see a marked change in their hair. The falling oestrogen levels can alter the texture of our hair and leave it dryer, more breakable and finer. Using products that are specifically formulated for dry and weak hair can help. Paying attention to your scalp health, which helps new hair to grow, is important, and be mindful of the heat tools you may use. All this can help improve texture and density.

You might also find that there is more hair on your face at this time and dark wiry hairs are appearing. Though your oestrogen levels are falling, you're producing the same amount of testosterone and that can result in things like coarse facial hair. Waxing these works well for many women but if you find they're growing too fast, speak to your doctor about topical reduction options, and laser and electrolysis treatments.

Incontinence

After pregnancy and childbirth, ageing has the biggest effect on our pelvic floor.

The pelvic floor is the supportive sling of muscles that work to protect our uterus, bladder and bowel, and oestrogen plays a part in keeping it healthy and working the way it should. As oestrogen levels drop, our pelvic floor strength can weaken. This can cause a number of issues or worsen any problems you may already have. These include:

- Urge incontinence: the sudden, very strong and frequent urge to go to the bathroom.
- Stress incontinence: urinating when you cough, laugh, sneeze or lift something.

- Nocturia: when you have to get up during the night to go to the bathroom.
- Urinary tract infections: some menopausal women are prone to getting more frequent UTIs. This is because as oestrogen levels fall, your vaginal tissue starts to thin, which makes it more prone to infection. Some women also have some difficulty fully emptying their bladder, which can also lead to infection.
- The post-menopausal oestrogen deficit influences the vaginal microbiome, reducing the number of lactobacilli in the vagina following the decrease in serum oestrogen levels. The relationship between the microbiome and post-menopausal vulvovaginal symptoms seems to be related to the bacterial vaginal population.

As well as incontinence, some women also experience vaginal problems like prolapse (which is a feeling of pressure, heaviness or a bulge coming down) and pain or decreased sensation when having sex.

Pelvic floor exercises
We are great at telling women what to do when it's slightly too late. We talk about osteoporosis at menopause and we tell women about pelvic floor exercises in antenatal classes. Why aren't we telling younger women about their bone health and explaining the importance of building up the pelvic floor before they are carrying an eight-pound baby inside them?

I would like to see pelvic floor health explained to girls in school. Why can't all muscle groups be spoken of the same way in PE? If we taught young women how to build a strong pelvic floor and made those exercises part of their lifelong fitness journey, I would see far fewer cases of stress incontinence and prolapse in my clinic.

A strong pelvic floor is a key part of women's health and one that is just not discussed often enough. The exercises aren't difficult, they can be done anywhere, and they make a huge difference. There are fantastic women's health physiotherapists who can help women who are already suffering but it would be another great aspect of women's health to normalise and shout about. We discuss men's prostates all the time very publicly now and there is absolutely no reason that a woman's pelvic floor cannot be the same.

There are two types of exercises to do – slow and fast – because there are two types of muscles in your pelvic floor: slow twitch muscles and fast twitch muscles.

Here's how to do the exercises:

- Sit in a comfortable position and make sure that your thighs, bottom and stomach are all relaxed. When you've got good at them you can do these exercises while walking, driving or exercising.
- Exhale before you begin and then tighten all the muscles in your back passage as if you are trying to stop yourself from breaking wind.
- When you have done this tighten and lift all the muscles in the front as if you are trying not to wee. Some people describe this as zipping up from your bottom to your urethra.
- Hold both sets of muscles for as long as you can while breathing in and out normally.
- The exercises can take a bit of getting used to and that's okay. Hold for as long as you can at the beginning and aim to eventually hold each exercise for 10 seconds.

- After each squeeze, relax for 10 seconds and start again. Try to do it 10 times.
- Now, the quick version. Breathe all the way out and do the same squeeze and lift motion but don't hold it this time. Relax, and do it again. Do these quick ones 20 times.

I have done an *Empowering Women* podcast with pelvic physiotherapist Elaine Barry that is free to download on my website. There is a great explanation of these exercises and a very helpful video on the HSE website.

Vaginal atrophy

The vaginal atrophy that we spoke about in the perimenopause chapter can continue to be an issue for some women in menopause. If you have a dry, uncomfortable feeling in this area, pain during sex, a burning sensation, itchiness, UTIs, changes to your urination or discharge, you may have vaginal atrophy.

Please don't be embarrassed about it or wait to speak to a doctor. It's a very normal perimenopause and menopause symptom and is just like any other issue you may need medical help with. I've seen some very sad cases of women living in pain because they were too mortified to seek help and that should never be the case.

Vaginal oestrogen pessaries work very well for this condition and can be taken twice a week. If you do not want to take pessaries, there are topical oestrogen creams that you can apply daily. HRT also helps.

It has been shown that vaginal oestrogens carry no increased risk of cancer reoccurrence among women undergoing treatment for breast cancer or those with a personal history of breast cancer.

Menopause and sex

There are many reasons why a woman may experience a low sex drive during menopause. The effects of low oestrogen on the vagina certainly have a part to play but so too does exhaustion and how women feel about themselves at this time. If we are feeling anxious, tired from all the things we have to do in life, have gained weight or are upset about how we're looking, sex can be the first thing to fall by the wayside.

Oestrogen creams and HRT can deal with vaginal problems like dryness and atrophy. Tiredness can be combated with lifestyle changes and HRT if it is needed for hot flushes. There are also treatments for muscle pain and restless legs. But a lot of what happens psychologically during menopause has to do with reclaiming and reframing this time in our lives. We should see it as an opportunity. Getting older is a positive thing.

Confidence, the freedom to travel and having time to spend with friends are some of the benefits of the advancing decades. If you have a family, with children growing up comes the opportunity for time alone with your partner and for things like new hobbies. It should be embraced, and we should be empowered to continue healthy sex lives.

Sex is also very good for stress levels and intimacy and as exercise!

It can be daunting and difficult to reclaim your sex life but one of the things we must keep doing is to communicate. Men need to know and understand what is going on, particularly around libido so that they can be supportive as well as not feel insecure and rejected. If you don't speak to your partner, they will not understand why you don't want to have sex. The first step should be a conversation.

Contraception

Speaking of sex, contraception is still very important both during perimenopause and for two years after menopause. Now, I want to preface what I'm going to say about contraception with a reiteration of my feelings about vasectomy and male responsibility. I cannot think of how to say it more strongly other than to repeat myself at every opportunity!

If you have completed your family and you have a male partner, please, please have a conversation about vasectomy. There is no reason for a woman to continue to take hormonal contraception when there are other options. It is, of course, totally fine if you have made that decision or want to manage irregular heavy periods with hormonal contraception, but if it is solely to prevent pregnancy you should certainly consider a vasectomy.

Vasectomy is a simple, quick and relatively painless operation (especially in comparison to what women deal with their entire lives) that would mean contraception is taken care of.

Though our fertility starts to decline from our mid-30s, if you're still having periods, even irregular ones, you may still be ovulating and are still fertile. If you want to avoid unplanned pregnancy during your perimenopausal and menopausal years, you will still have to think about contraception.

You will be familiar with the combined oral contraceptive pill which contains both oestrogen and progesterone. We don't recommend the use of this in women over the age of 40 so it is usually not prescribed in this age group.

The mini pill or progesterone-only pill is a popular option for women in this category, as it can be taken for as long as contraception is needed, so right up to menopause, and can help with heavy periods.

The other type of progesterone-based contraception is the Mirena coil, which contains a small amount of progesterone that is released gradually. It can be used for both contraception and as the progesterone component of HRT (alongside an oestrogen patch, cream or gel). It is changed every five years.

The contraceptive implant is like the Mirena coil in that it releases progesterone slowly. It is inserted under the skin of the upper arm and is changed every three years.

There is also barrier method contraception (condoms) and vasectomy. Some doctors may speak to you about tubal ligation, which you will already know I do not recommend.

Osteoporosis

This is a bone disease that affects 80% of women during and after menopause, weakening our bones and making us more at risk of unexpected fractures. It's often called a silent disease because there are no symptoms until that first break. But there are ways of preventing osteoporosis and of slowing down the rate of bone loss that you may already have.

Because the ratio of bone build-up and bone loss is impaired by this disease, the bone becomes more porous and brittle. This often results in hip fracture, but can also damage other typical weak spots such as the pelvis, spine and lower arm. Hip fractures can be associated with immobility and thus a higher instance of pulmonary embolisms and sometimes mortality.

More than half of patients who develop osteoporosis will suffer a broken bone within the space of four years.

The three warning signs of osteoporosis are back pain, loss of height and a stooped posture.

Risk factors for osteoporosis

- Being female
- Being over 65
- Hyperthyroidism
- Overactive parathyroid and adrenal glands
- Low levels of oestrogen (as in menopause)
- Treatments for prostate cancer that reduce testosterone levels in men and treatments for breast cancer that reduce oestrogen levels in women; both accelerate bone loss

- Family history
- Body frame – women with a smaller frame are at a higher risk
- Low calcium intake
- Coeliac disease
- Gastrointestinal surgery
- Long-term steroid use
- Sedentary lifestyle
- Excessive alcohol consumption
- Smoking

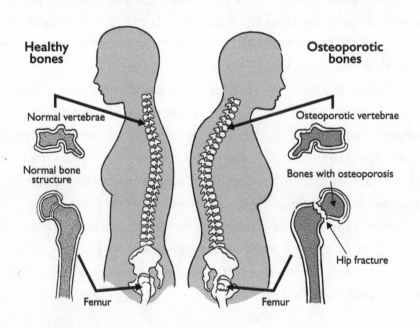

Healthy bones

Osteoporotic bones

Normal vertebrae

Osteoporotic vertebrae

Normal bone structure

Bones with osteoporosis

Hip fracture

Femur

Femur

Menopause

As you might expect, we're back to oestrogen again. It protects your bones and there is a direct link between osteoporosis and low levels of oestrogen in perimenopause and menopause.

A good way to find out how your bones are doing is with a bone density scan, which you may know as a DEXA scan. The results will give you a T-score. A value of -1SD is normal, -1 to -2.5 shows some bone loss, which is called osteopenia (the stage before osteoporosis – it does not necessarily become osteoporosis), and below -2.5 is osteoporosis.

If you are at risk of osteoporosis, there are some things you should be doing to mitigate your risk of developing it:

- Take regular exercise, particularly weight-bearing and muscle-strengthening exercises.
- Eat a diet rich in calcium and vitamin D. Make sure your vitamin D levels are adequate by asking your GP to check them. We each need to take 1000mg of calcium per day.
- Reduce the amount of alcohol you drink.
- Stop smoking.

If you do have osteoporosis, there is a range of very good medications that your doctor can prescribe. What is most important is that we no longer see the 'dowager's hump' that was so common in post-menopausal women in the past as they were not treated. It is very important that you get a regular DEXA and that you look after your bone health.

CASE HISTORY: ANNE MARIE

Anne Marie came to me with severe back pain; she was 56 at the time. She had had her ovaries and uterus removed at 46 and went into sudden menopause. Unfortunately, she was not given HRT. I see this all too often. Because of that lack of HRT she now had severe osteoporosis, a vertebral fracture in her fourth lumbar vertebra and had lost significant height, which she was very upset about.

I treated her with parathyroid hormone for her osteoporosis, checked her vitamin D levels and restored them, and gave her diet advice and bone-strengthening exercises. She did well but a lot of her problems and suffering could have been prevented if she had been given HRT after her hysterectomy.

Your body, weight and the menopause

With everything that's changing it's no wonder that the shape of your body will too. Women often find that they're suddenly putting on weight around their tummy in their perimenopausal and menopausal years.

There's a combination of reasons for this. The body needs energy for the monthly growth of the egg and ovulation as well as the transformation of the follicle into the corpus luteum. From the age of 35 onwards, anovulatory cycles become more frequent.

Progesterone is responsible for the fact that the body temperature goes up 0.5 degrees in the latter half of the cycle. If this temperature rise fails to take place then the energy which is otherwise required for heat production is not used up.

After menopause women burn 300 fewer calories per day. I think it is very important that women know this so they can stop the self-blame game that women are always doing to themselves.

The other factor is that women over 40 exercise less than they used to. In menopause, falling DHEA (a steroid hormone that your body converts into oestrogen) levels inhibit muscle build-up; remember, muscle is our best fat burner. Resistance to leptin, one of the hunger hormones that helps to balance your natural appetite, often develops at this time. Physical activity is the best way to make the receptors responsive again and reduce the hunger pangs; exercise and healthy eating help to reactivate the feelings of satiety.

Oestrogen dominance leads to water retention and a redistribution of fat around the abdominal area. As I said earlier, the lack of progesterone affects thyroid production and the thyroid can no longer control the production of oestrogen.

Recent studies have found that toxins in the environment and in microplastics are responsible for profound disturbances in our hormonal system. These endocrine disrupters interfere with the satiety hormones and the storage and breaking down of fat cells.

Scientists also believe that vitamin D sends out signals for fat burning, deciding whether or not fat will be burned for energy by directing vitamin D receptors to fat cells. If fat is not used for energy, it is stored in the abdomen or on the hips.

A famous American study was the first to prove the importance of intestinal flora to body weight. When the intestinal flora of overweight mice was transplanted into the mice of normal weight, these latter mice became overweight despite being on a diet. Swedish scientists proved that overweight people have less varied intestinal flora and also more bacteria that metabolise special carbohydrates in their intestines.

Overweight people often have fewer bacteria of the strain *Bacteroides* and more of the strain *Firmicutes*. The good news is that the composition of the intestinal flora can be actively controlled through a good diet. Fermented products, probiotics and prebiotics ensure a balanced microbiome and this helps to regulate weight.

Hormonal changes play a part but so too does fatigue and the comfort eating that comes with that. Our metabolism slows down around perimenopause and menopause and the way that fat is stored and distributed in our bodies also changes. Where you may have been a pear shape and carried any extra weight around your hips and thighs, in these years that may shift up to your stomach area. This is called an apple shape and it's not only hard for lots of women psychologically, but it's also not very good for your health.

A larger waist puts you at a higher risk of heart disease and can also mean a bigger risk of Type 2 diabetes. You can be an apple shape and not overweight but still at a higher risk of heart disease, diabetes and cancer. It's very important to monitor the weight around your stomach area. You may have previously got away with your sweet tooth, but you won't once your metabolism slows down – the fat will all go to your abdomen.

The fat cells around your tummy are very metabolically active; they're an active endocrine organ and people forget that. Those fat cells produce six active hormones around the abdomen that damage the arteries.

I do not believe in strict diets; rather, moderation is the key to getting everything under control. The Mediterranean diet is still the best model. That basically means lots of fresh vegetables, fruits and fish. Hydration is also very important, so make sure to get your 2 litres per day.

If you have a sweet tooth, have a square of really good dark chocolate instead of something more sugary. I always say that your problems start in the trolley, so don't put the treats in there in the first place. You're fooling yourself if you say you're buying them for the rest of the family. If you keep the fridge and the presses healthy, you'll stay healthy too. The good news is that 80% of your weight can be influenced by your lifestyle.

Cardiovascular disease and menopause

Menopause itself does not cause heart disease but it does increase certain risk factors around getting it.

Oestrogen has a big protectant factor from heart disease for women, but as we age and our oestrogen levels fall so too does that protection. After menopause women are just as likely as men to have a heart attack. In fact, in Ireland, cardiovascular disease, particularly heart attack and stroke, is one of the biggest killers of women. Many women worry about breast cancer, but according to the Irish Heart Foundation you are six times more likely to die from cardiovascular disease.

Smoking, obesity, high blood pressure, high cholesterol, a family history of heart disease, being sedentary and having diabetes all put you at increased risk of heart disease.

Women of menopausal age should have their blood pressure, cholesterol and blood sugar levels checked. HRT offers some protection against heart disease in early menopause but that ceases when you stop taking it at around 60.

The best course of action is to know the risks and mind your health. A good diet, exercise, reducing your alcohol intake and lowering your stress levels all help reduce your chances of cardiovascular disease.

Exercise

I believe that diet and exercise should work hand in hand. There's no point in being thin and very weak. Instead, I want to see women maintain their weight but be fit and strong and able to do all the things they could before.

Muscle mass decreases continuously from the age of 30 by 5% per decade. So by the age of 50, you have 10% less muscle than when you were 30. Therefore, it's important to rebuild and maintain muscle mass with exercise. Remember that muscle is our main fat burner. Muscles are the biggest consumers of calories alongside our brains.

I recommend that women do some muscle-building exercises three times a week. Make sure the weights are right for your body, so discuss this with your physiotherapist or trainer. Remember that it's important to pace yourself and don't sacrifice your rest by getting up at 6 a.m. to try to fit this into your day. Find a time that suits you and tell your family you're setting aside that time for your health.

Exercise of any kind supports the metabolism and keeps insulin at a steady level. Our metabolism slows down at the age of 40, particularly when our muscle mass decreases, which causes our bodies to lose their best ally for the direct consumption of carbohydrates. Exercise can also restore leptin to the right level and therefore normalise the feeling of hunger and help weight loss.

Do exercise that supports your core and your back so that it doesn't become a problem in the future. Strengthen your limbs and practise flexibility. Regular exercise, even walking for 30 minutes a day, reduces the hot flushing, muscle pain, insomnia and weight gain many menopausal women experience. It also promotes bone formation and protects against osteoporosis, all cardiovascular diseases and almost all cancers. Regular exercise has been shown to reduce the risk of breast cancer.

Exercise also increases our serotonin levels so you're literally doing something that will make you happy!

Types of exercise

You want to do two things here. You want to protect, build and maintain your muscles and bone density and you want to keep your heart healthy.

You can run or, if that is not for you, you can go for some great brisk walks. These will build your stamina and give your heart a workout. Really walk now, I'm not talking about a stroll with a big coffee in hand. It has to be a workout. The recommendation is that we do at least 150 minutes of exercise over seven days.

For strength training, you can do classes with weights or kettlebells (lots of local gyms or community centres run great classes that aren't intimidating at all) or you can take up yoga or Pilates, which use your own body weight to make you stronger. Anyone who says that yoga and Pilates are easy workouts and are very gentle has never done it for long – your first introductory class may be very nice and easy but the longer you go, the harder it gets and they're a great workout.

Benefits of exercise

- It lowers the risk of cardiovascular disease.
- It lowers blood sugar as the sugar is removed from the blood and burned.
- It regulates insulin and prevents insulin resistance.
- It stimulates bone formation and maintains bone density.
- Regular exercise has been proven to reduce the risk of colon and breast cancer.
- It improves concentration and memory.
- It helps with brain fog.
- It stimulates the formation of the small power plants in the body, the mitochondria in the cells, as well as many repair and growth processes.
- It increases your levels of serotonin, which is your happy hormone.
- It helps delay ageing. Cell inflammation and cell breakdown have been shown to be delayed by regular exercise.

Menopause through cancer

If you have reached menopause because of a cancer diagnosis and treatment, my heart goes out to you. It can be so hard that on top of being told that you have cancer, you must then go through menopause sooner than you would expect to.

Some cancer treatments, though not all, cause early menopause, including hysterectomy that includes the removal of the ovaries, radiotherapy to the pelvis, hormone therapy and chemotherapy. Your oncologist will be able to tell you if your menopause is temporary or permanent.

Living through the symptoms of menopause while also trying to get better after your diagnosis can be very tough.

Your oncology team will liaise with your doctor and they are best placed to help alleviate those symptoms. Bringing them a diary of what you have been experiencing can be a good idea. Some of the symptoms of menopause can be very similar to the symptoms you may get from your treatment and so communication is very important.

How do you communicate?

Menopause isn't just about you, it's about everyone around you too. It's how you react to them and how they react to you when you are in need of support, love and, let's face it, help!

You are self-aware but your partner and teenage children probably are not and so it's our job (yes, another job for us!) to talk to them about it. Our society, up until recently, lived in a state of near blissful ignorance about what goes on around menopause. But if we have only informed society of the bare minimum about menopause and perimenopause, how can we expect them to be well informed? They don't know why we're bleeding more than usual, why we can't sleep, why we're emotional or angry, and if we want their kindness, we must explain it.

They're not the only ones we need to communicate with.

Biology is a wonderful thing, and the timing of menopause means that many of us are in the midst of symptoms just as our children are finding their way through puberty. That can make for some explosive standoffs! But teens are remarkable and an honest conversation about how you're both going through hormonal changes and that your moods are affected just as much as theirs will go a long way to creating a peaceful home. A little understanding of each other is a great thing.

It might feel awkward at first, but remember that you need their help; what is happening is normal, and if you don't do this you will continue to suffer in silence, and who has the time or patience for that?

Liveline with Joe Duffy

I have been doing lectures on hormones and menopause for about eight years. I have organised three empowerment conferences to date at the University of Limerick and lots of podcasts to educate women on their hormonal health. In the process, I could see that the more I spoke the more the narrative was changing. Women were being empowered and educated and it was wonderful. It was giving women a platform to speak out. The media started picking up on that and I was getting calls from journalists for articles.

It was at this point that the researcher on *Liveline* contacted me and asked me to come on and talk to Joe Duffy, which of course I was delighted to do.

There was such an outpouring from callers on that one show that they had to keep it going; one day clearly wasn't enough and so it became a whole week. I think they were very surprised. I was not. I had heard all these stories before (they were the reason that Lorraine Keane and I had travelled the country educating women about menopause). They couldn't get over the number of women who were ringing in and crying, talking about the horrendous suffering they had gone through and the lack of people listening to them. It really was horrific. It was very sad to hear how they were being treated so poorly. Some of them had lost a good 15 years of their life, which is dreadful.

One woman phoned in complaining of restless legs and I explained that it was a big symptom of menopause. Then more women phoned in with the same thing and I realised that, while hot flushes and night sweats were known about, other symptoms like restless legs and brain fog were not.

The number of women calling in who didn't sleep as a result of having restless legs was shocking to me. A lot of them hadn't slept for 10 years. There's no reason for them to suffer like that and they were putting themselves at risk of hormonal imbalance and immune dysfunction as a result.

The beauty of that week, though, was the huge listenership. Women felt empowered to talk about menopause. Now that other women had shared their stories, they knew there was no taboo and they felt compelled to share their own stories and talk about them. Support groups were set up and women finally felt relieved to share their hormonal journey.

So many men were reached – taxi drivers, farmers, office workers – and all heard the suffering that women were going through. I couldn't believe the reaction from men. It was phenomenal and so moving. You could clearly see how vital it is that men understand what happens so that they can be supportive.

CASE HISTORY: MIRIAM

In my career, I've come across some really difficult cases of menopause. When Miriam came to see me she had some very severe symptoms and was really struggling. She had very frequent bouts of hot flushes, she wasn't sleeping and was exhausted, she had restless legs at night, brain fog and very severe headaches.

She had been to see her GP who had diagnosed her with depression and prescribed anti-depressants. She was very upset with that and believed she wasn't depressed. She was a very positive person, a mother of three children and a hard-working farmer.

Despite her obvious difficulties, her husband was not supportive and kept calling her in the morning to get up to work even though she had only got to sleep at 6 a.m. because of all her night-time symptoms. He had no understanding of menopause and thought that she was using it as an excuse to be lazy. He kept saying that it was better for her not to lie down, she should just keep going instead.

Miriam had suffered terribly for 10 years. Interestingly, she had had very heavy periods from puberty and I often find a lot of women with heavy periods have more severe menopause, most probably because the hormone control centre is tired coming into it.

After examining Miriam, I explained all the symptoms to her. I also rang her husband and spoke to him about what his wife was going through so that he could understand that she needed to rest until her hormone control centre was recharged.

She started on HRT and treatment for peripheral nerve pain and her symptoms began to subside. She was thrilled three months later when I saw her again as she had energy for the first time in a long time, she was sleeping every night and the brain fog had lifted. Most important, her husband now understood what was happening and her need for rest.

CASE HISTORY: MARGARET

When Margaret made an appointment to see me she was 47. Her periods had stopped, she had severe restless legs and hadn't slept in a year. She had brain fog and terrible vaginal dryness and she was very temperamental, which she said was unusual for her.

She was finding it really hard to cope with her teenage children because they weren't helping out and she was exhausted from looking after them and clearing up their mess.

She couldn't make love with her husband because of the vaginal dryness. Whenever I can I always speak to a couple together about menopause. It is so important that the partner understands what's going on so that they can be supportive. Margaret's husband was in the waiting room that day but if he hadn't been I would have rung him.

I spoke to them both about the hormonal imbalance Margaret was experiencing due to menopause and about the complete and utter exhaustion she was trying to live through as a result.

I asked her husband to make a rota for himself and the children to help around the house. Women are not slaves to their husbands or children and it's vital that everyone plays their part at home. It also empowers children to be able to look after themselves in the future

I then set to work on Margaret's physical symptoms, starting with vaginal dryness. No woman should suffer that, and we opted for oestrogen pessaries that women can use twice a week and are very safe. I also prescribed Estradot, a bio-identical oestrogen patch, twice a week, and micronised progesterone. As you know by now, progesterone helps with sleep as well as keeping the balance correct with oestrogen to prevent endometrial proliferation.

Speaking up

Well-known women being vocal about their experience of menopause is vital. It gives a voice to a natural part of womanhood that has for too long been shrouded in mystery and embarrassment.

I have done so much work in my Hormone Health lectures with Lorraine Keane, who generously gave her time to speak about her own experience. She also shared her journey of perimenopause, which began early for her, and it empowered women to talk to her.

Internationally, some huge names have started to become more vocal too, which is just wonderful to see.

Michelle Obama

In the summer of 2020, the former First Lady of the USA spoke about menopause on her Spotify podcast, speaking to gynaecologist Sharon Malone. 'I have a very healthy baseline, and also, well, I was experiencing hormone shifts because of infertility, having to take shots and all that,' Obama explained. 'I experienced the night sweats, even in my 30s, and when you think of the other symptoms that come along, just hot flashes, I mean, I had a few before I started taking hormones.'

She even spoke about having hot flushes at very inopportune times, like on Marine One, the presidential helicopter. 'I remember having one on Marine One. I'm dressed, I need to get out, walk into an event, and literally, it was like somebody put a furnace in my core and turned it on high, and then everything started melting. And I thought, well, this is crazy – I can't, I can't, I can't do this.'

She also said her husband was unfazed by what was happening to her and other women he worked with and took it in his stride. 'He didn't fall apart because he found out there were several women in his staff that were going through menopause. It was just sort of like, "Oh, well, turn the air conditioner on."'

Oprah Winfrey

Oprah Winfrey has also spoken about her menopause symptoms. She wrote about them in her magazine, O, in 2019. 'For two years I didn't sleep well. Never a full night. No peace. Restlessness and heart palpitations were my steady companions at nightfall. This was back when I was 48 to 50. I went to see a cardiologist. Took medication. Wore a heart monitor for weeks. And then one day, walking through the offices of *The Oprah Winfrey Show*, I picked up a copy of *The Wisdom of Menopause*, Dr Christiane Northrup's book, and the pages fell open to the heading "Palpitations: Your Heart's Wake-Up Call". I took it as a sign.

'Contained in that book was the answer I'd been going doctor to doctor trying to figure out. Until that point in my adult life, I don't recall one serious conversation with another woman about what to expect.'

Oprah took menopause as an opportunity to focus on herself. 'So many women I've talked to see menopause as a blessing. I've discovered that this is your moment to reinvent yourself after years of focusing on the needs of everyone else.'

Gwyneth Paltrow

Gwyneth Paltrow, Oscar-winning actress and founder of Goop, wants to 'brand' menopause in a new way. Speaking on the Goop platform in 2018 she said: 'I think when you get into perimenopause, you notice a lot of changes. I can feel the hormonal shifts happening, the sweating, the moods – you're all of a sudden furious for no reason. Menopause gets a really bad rap and needs a bit of rebranding. I remember when my mother went through menopause and it was such a big deal, and I think there was grief around it for her and all these emotions. I don't think we have in our society a great example of an aspirational menopausal woman.'

Gillian Anderson

The actress, who stars in *Sex Education* and *The Crown*, has spoken about going through early menopause for years. She told *People* magazine in 2017 that she'd love the shame around the subject to disappear. 'How wonderful would it be if we could get to a place where we are able to have these conversations openly and without shame? Admit, freely, that this is what's going on. So we don't feel like we're going mad or insane or alone in any of the symptoms we are having. Perimenopause and menopause should be treated as the rites of passage that they are. If not celebrated, then at least accepted and acknowledged and honoured.'

Emma Thompson

When Emma Thompson was promoting her film *Late Night*, about a female chat show host in her 50s, she told *BBC Breakfast*: 'I've never regarded menopause as a taboo. Although of course, you don't realise until you mention it and suddenly everyone goes, thank God you're talking about it, you don't realise that it has, in fact, been side-lined, and not discussed because, of course, it's something to do with women who have been side-lined and not discussed for centuries. So, as we are coming out as it were from this oppression, it's very interesting to see our reactions to things that we know are there, but that men don't, because they haven't seen it, which is why it's lovely when men react to this film and love it.'

CASE HISTORY: JULIE

We don't speak too much about the bowel and menopause. Julie, 59, had experienced IBS ever since menopause. She had been biopsied, had bloods taken and had scopes and all were normal. She also had restless legs and peripheral neuropathy. She had tried specialist diets and none had worked. It had been going on for years and she was exhausted from it.

I knew that HRT alone would not address these issues. I have seen a lot of this in patients with perimenopause and menopause and it comes down to hormones. Remember, hormones control the muscles and when there is a hormonal imbalance the circadian rhythm is off. In some women, this leads to bowel issues.

Some patients get IBS mid-cycle and with their period. In endocrinology we are used to dealing with peripheral neuropathy and autonomic neuropathy in diabetic patients and this was a form of the same thing. Thankfully, Julie responded very well to the treatment.

The dietitian put her on a low FODMAP diet, which cuts out certain carbohydrates. I treated her with Gabapentin to treat the restless legs, and this combination improved her bowel symptoms.

Her husband rang me personally to thank me for having his wife back and her son wrote from New York to thank me for giving his mother's life back as she had been suffering so dreadfully. It is so lovely to be able to make a positive difference in someone's life. This is why I became a doctor in the first place.

CASE HISTORY: URSULA

When Ursula came to me she was 53 years old and was going through menopause. She had been put on HRT by her GP but her main issue was severe anxiety that had only started when menopause hit.

Her husband who had come to the appointment with her said she was a completely different person. She was normally calm and controlled but was now constantly anxious and they were both very concerned. It was affecting her personal and professional life.

This is quite common in menopause, and I explained the reasons for it. Knowing what's normal is very important and a lot of women are reassured when they know they are not losing it and that what they are experiencing is normal and can be sorted.

HRT is great for so many symptoms of menopause. Sometimes we need to add in additional medications if the patient is very anxious, such as Gabapentin or Amytriptaline, as these also work on peripheral nerves and restore hormone balance

Ursula did very well with treatment, but I shudder to think what happened to women many years ago who suffered in this way. I have heard so many stories of women who were institutionalised after menopause and never saw their families again. Women's mental health was poorly looked after in the past and women with menopause-related depression and anxiety were sometimes committed to asylums instead of being treated. In Victorian times doctors believed that the uterus and the brain were connected and that women in menopause had a condition called climacteric insanity.

CASE HISTORY: KATE

When Kate came to see me at the age of 52, she had menopausal symptoms and severe urticaria, which is a raised bumpy rash. When I explained how the two were connected, she was thrilled because she thought she was losing it. So many women are so relieved when they understand what is going on.

In this case, as well as prescribing HRT, I also gave Kate an antihistamine. Mast cells are immune cells that release prostaglandin and histamine. Histamine causes swelling when there is inflammation (urticaria) but also controls libido and stomach acid and stimulates the brain. Histamine also releases excess oestrogen production and uterine mast cells release prostaglandins and heparin, which can directly cause heavy bleeding.

I advised Kate to get more rest. I have to lecture so many women about this. When your body is going through a hormonal change you must rest to be able to deal with the change.

So many women are so disempowered compared to men that they feel they should be active all the time. Kate was getting up at 6 a.m. to make lunches for her adolescent children, who were more than capable of doing it themselves, then going to work all day, was secretary of a local GAA club, loved a clean house and never delegated to her spouse or kids. As a doctor, I can prescribe all the treatments in the world but it has to go hand in hand with women empowering themselves to make lifestyle changes, loving themselves, putting boundaries in place and learning to say the word 'No'. A psychologist once told me that women work too hard in the home in order to prove themselves as a 'supermum' and thus keep themselves visible when they are not visible to themselves. This is something that we will discuss later.

Hormone replacement therapy

HRT is considered the gold standard of treatment for symptoms of menopause. Women who have their uterus still intact will need oestrogen and progesterone replaced, while women who have had a hysterectomy will only need oestrogen.

The reason you need both oestrogen and progesterone if you still have your uterus is that the oestrogen is needed to treat the symptoms of menopause while the progesterone is there to protect the lining of your uterus from endometrial cancer. Oestrogen without progesterone increases the risk of endometrial/uterine cancer.

Generally, you give HRT for the shortest amount of time you can, and you stop it at 60. HRT is now considered a very safe medicine but there are risks associated with everything in life and you must weigh them against the benefits. The benefits of HRT usually outweigh the risks for most women.

There is still a lot of fear around HRT. Most of it is unnecessary and it can be a lifeline for many women who are suffering from debilitating symptoms that have an impact on their day-to-day lives. The fear mainly comes from a study conducted by the Women's Health Initiative in the USA that ran from 1993 to 2002. In that time, they studied over 16,000 women in the States, giving half of them HRT and the other half a placebo. The results of the study were catastrophic and showed an increase in heart disease and breast cancer in those given HRT. In the years afterwards, the prescription rate for HRT fell by 70%. In 2016, the scientists behind the study apologised for a misinterpretation of their data. There has been a lot more research done since this study, and we now know a lot more about the benefits and risks of HRT. There are different HRT products on the market now and many doctors, including myself, will prescribe a HRT patch which means you're receiving the hormones transdermally – through the skin – so there is no increase in the risk of blood clots.

Benefits of HRT

- The primary benefit of HRT is that it reduces or relieves most menopausal symptoms including hot flushes, night sweats, vaginal dryness, low libido, brain fog and mood swings. It is the most effective treatment for the symptoms of menopause and perimenopause.
- It is also beneficial for osteoporosis, which is more common after menopause and can help prevent thinning of the bones.
- It can ease an overactive bladder and the need to go to the toilet frequently.
- It can lower your risk of heart disease provided you start it within 10 years of menopause.

- Women who use HRT are at a lower risk of developing Type 2 diabetes.
- The risk of bowel cancer is reduced by half when women take HRT for 9 to 14 years.

Risks of HRT

- Stroke: there is a small increase in the risk of stroke but for women under 60 that risk is generally very low.
- Cardiovascular disease: HRT does not significantly increase the risk of cardiovascular disease (including heart disease and stroke) if it is started before 60. In fact, it may reduce your risk.
- Blood clots: HRT tablets can increase the risk of blood clots, but it is considered a small risk. If you take HRT patches or gels, there is no increased risk of clots.
- Breast cancer: combined HRT (with both oestrogen and progesterone) can be associated with a small increase in the risk of breast cancer. That risk is linked to how long you take it and falls again immediately after you stop taking it. There's very little or no change at all in the risk of breast cancer if you are on oestrogen-only HRT.
- Endometrial cancer: if you have your uterus and haven't had a hysterectomy you need to take combined HRT. Oestrogen without progesterone increases the risk of endometrial/ uterine cancer.

Types of HRT

There are different types of HRT available, and I always discuss the options with my patients. The two main hormones used in HRT are oestrogen (the types used here include oestradiol, oestrone and oestriol) and progesterone, either a synthetic version or a micronised progesterone which is sometimes called natural or bio-identical progesterone and is chemically identical to the hormone we produce naturally.

In HRT you either take both of these hormones together, which is called combined HRT, or oestrogen on its own, which is called oestrogen-only HRT. The oestrogen-only version is only recommended if you have had your uterus removed.

As well as different types of HRT there are different ways of taking it.

Tablets

Taking HRT in tablet form is one of the most common ways of taking it. The tablets are usually taken once a day and both types of HRT are available in this form. There are some risks associated with the tablet version of HRT, such as blood clots, but the overall risk is still very low.

Skin patches

This is another common way of taking HRT and one that many women prefer. You stick the patch to your skin and replace it every few days. Using the patches avoids some of the side effects of tablets (like indigestion) and because you're receiving the hormones transdermally they do not increase the risk of blood clots. Both types of HRT are available in patch form.

Oestrogen gel

This is becoming a very popular form of HRT. You rub the gel into your skin once a day and it does not increase the risk of blood clots. If you still have your uterus, you will also need to take some form of progesterone because of the risk of uterine cancer when taking oestrogen only.

Vaginal oestrogen

If you have vaginal dryness but no other symptoms, you may want to try an oestrogen cream, pessary or ring. There is no increased risk of breast cancer with this and so you do not have to take progesterone with it even if you still have a uterus.

How and when

The way you take your HRT will depend on where you are in your perimenopause/menopause journey. There are two types of routines available: cyclical and continuous.

Cyclical HRT is most often recommended for women who have menopausal symptoms but still have their periods. There are two types of cyclical HRT – monthly and three-monthly. You can either take oestrogen every day and progesterone for the second half of your cycle or you can take oestrogen daily and progesterone with it for 14 days every three months. Monthly HRT is recommended for those women who still have regular periods and three-monthly is usually for women who have more irregular cycles.

Continuous HRT is recommended for women who have reached menopause. Combined HRT is taken every day without a break in this routine.

It's recommended to take HRT for the shortest amount of time feasible. Although some women do continue to take HRT after 60, most doctors don't recommend its use after this age as most menopausal symptoms will have passed. I have come across several women who still had severe hot flushes in their sixth and seventh decade so they could not come off HRT, but we had to monitor their hearts closely and do regular mammograms. Also, if you are coming off HRT, you need to taper oestrogen down slowly over weeks or even months to shelter you from oestrogen withdrawal symptoms. You can stop the progesterone at any time because it does not cause withdrawal effects

Testosterone is sometimes prescribed to enhance libido and clitoral sensitivity, and it works, but only if oestrogen therapy is already in place. However, we need more research into this area for women. There have been some studies showing it promotes insulin resistance. It is probably okay to try a small dose of testosterone so long as you also take oestradiol and progesterone to shelter you from high androgens, but more research in this area is needed and we need to see more safety data.

CHAPTER SEVEN
Diet and Hormones

It starts with the supermarket shop. If you find it hard to resist, do not buy it. Don't say you're buying it for the family or to keep it in a treat press – literally don't put it in your trolley. It's a vicious circle. If it's there, you'll eat it, especially if you're tired. Nobody in the house needs the junk.

Everyone is different

At this point, I would like to say that I know that everyone is different. I absolutely do not think that everyone should be 10 stone and a neat size 10. The world is made up of billions of people, every one of them a different size and shape. I don't think that anyone's experience of medical

---

care should be different because of their size and I'm sorry if you have experienced that. However, I will say that it's important for everyone to pay attention to where they carry their weight because that does have an impact on our hormonal health.

Hormones and weight, diet and metabolism

Several hormones influence our appetite, distribution of body fat and our metabolism. They include leptin, insulin, oestrogen, androgen and the growth hormone. The balance of hormones, our diet, exercise and rest all work together in our body and when one is out of kilter it can change the way they all function. This explains why you crave sugar or carbs when you're tired or stressed.

Leptin is made by fat cells and is released into the bloodstream. It works by reducing your appetite and telling your body that it's full and doesn't need more food. Oestrogen and androgen play a big part in the distribution of body fat, which in turn plays a big role in the development of conditions like heart disease and stroke. A major factor in these conditions is abdominal weight. I am always talking about the importance of not putting on weight around your middle or becoming what some people call apple-shaped. Women who have reached menopause don't produce as much oestrogen as they used to which, as well as everything else that happens, can affect metabolism, causing it to slow, and lead to abdominal weight gain.

It is so important during perimenopause and menopause to watch our diets and make sure that we're keeping an eye on portion size and sugar and getting enough fibre.

Diabetes

If we're talking about diet and weight and hormones we must talk again about diabetes or actually about the pre-diabetic stage that we call metabolic syndrome. We need more education about metabolic syndrome, which is where you get fatty liver, insulin resistance, high or higher levels of LDL (the bad cholesterol) and hypertension.

There is an epidemic of Type 2 diabetes now that is a big concern. I have been working with diabetic patients since I started my medical career, and I see many women presenting with Type 2 diabetes because of weight.

People need to understand that if we get the people who are at the pre-diabetic stage to lose weight, focus on their diet and get healthy we can actually reverse diabetes completely – it won't turn into Type 2 diabetes. And it is that abdominal weight in particular that needs to be addressed.

But if you don't get it early people can develop diabetes that's not reversible with any amount of lifestyle changes, the pancreas is damaged and that's it.

You see stories on TV and online about amazing 800-calorie diets that can reverse diabetes, but the reality is none of us can maintain life on just 800 calories a day. I would see this a lot in patients who have had gastric bypasses. They do great and they reverse their diabetes for about four years, but then once they go back to eating the way they did before, their diabetes comes back. That's the reality.

The problem with metabolic syndrome is that you don't necessarily know that you're at that stage. The only visible marker would be that you have abdominal obesity. You might also have high blood pressure, but that's silent and you might not get the headaches that sometimes come with it.

There's no excessive thirst, you're not going to the toilet frequently, and you're not exhausted yet. Unless you've had your lipids checked, you wouldn't know that you had high LDL and low HDL cholesterol.

That's why we need education about diabetes. People need to understand what that fat around their middle is potentially causing. People often think I'm just banging a weight loss drum, but Type 2 diabetes is at a critical level in this country and I want everyone to know what they can do to protect themselves from it.

The reason it's so important is that, yes, it's a terrible health condition to have, but the economic cost of diabetes is huge. In 2018 Diabetes Ireland said that the current cost of managing diabetes was estimated to be 12–14% (approximately €2 billion) of the annual health budget, with very little of this spent on the prevention or effective self-management of diabetes.

That's a huge amount of money and Diabetes Ireland expects it to keep rising. There are associated conditions like retinopathy, kidney disease, nerve damage and surgeries for limb amputations that add to those costs. In addition, 75% of patients with Type 2 diabetes will get heart disease. There are enormous economic and health factors to consider, which is why I believe that we need to concentrate on this health crisis a great deal more.

I feel very strongly about the role that diet plays in hormonal health. It is all linked. From what you eat and when, to how much water you consume, every single mouthful has an impact on your hormones.

Diet and Hormones

There are a lot of diets out there that claim to cure you of illnesses and diseases and promise dramatic weight loss, but for me, diet and hormones boil down to one quite simple word: moderation. I do acknowledge, however, that there are also genetic causes of weight gain and there are now treatments for those patients.

What I always suggest is a very simple diet of three healthy meals a day and two snacks. I see a lot of patients who want to lose more weight or take things to an extreme, but all the research has shown that though they lose weight initially, they won't stick to it. I think it's because as a human being, you can only do an extreme diet for so long; none of us can adhere to it for ever. Also, these really strict diets can do damage to other organs, and we don't want that.

It's much easier to stick to a simple plan of three meals, two snacks and plenty of hydration. Have a variety of food types on your plate, make sure they are the right portion sizes and keep your intake of sugar low. Dietitians advise eating 'all the colours of the rainbow'.

Don't be too restrictive either; allow space for treats in your life. The more you tell yourself you can't have something the more you'll want it and you'll end up bingeing, then restricting again and beating yourself up about it. It's a yo-yo effect, which isn't good.

Portion size is important too. Have a look at the literal size of your plate. A lot of people are fooling themselves and eating off huge serving platters. You are harming no one but yourself.

Don't cook for leftovers either. I remember when I was in Trinity there was a great doctor who used to talk about our famine genes. He used to say that if you're cooking dinner, you should only put in the number of potatoes that you need. If you cook extra, you won't leave them because it's inherent in our genetic make-up that we can't leave food behind. If you end up with leftovers, wonderful, they make great healthy lunches, but if you regularly plan for leftovers and find you have none, you know exactly where all that extra food is going.

Try to just take it back to healthy basics. Specific diets that are low carb or high protein may get the balance in your body wrong and other organs will suffer. Eat natural food, choose a mix of fruit and vegetables, limit the amount of processed food you eat and drink alcohol in moderation.

Sit down to eat; don't pick off the kids' plates or stand and eat something in a hurry because you're so busy. Treat yourself like a person and have your dinner. Prioritise your health and your happiness. Do not skip breakfast, which is the most important meal of the day and kicks off your metabolism for the day. A lot of women skip breakfast while looking after their children. This is bad for you and also bad mentorship for the children who need to see you looking after yourself so that they will do it in their adulthood.

The gut, the bowel, the microbiome and your hormones

A lot has been said recently about the brain–gut axis. Having good gut health is crucial for good brain health and cognitive function. It is a two-way system of communication that links the emotional and cognitive centres in the brain with the gut. I have had the privilege of being lectured to by Professor Ted Dinan as a student at Trinity College Dublin. Professor Dinan coined the word 'psychobiotics', a term describing how bacteria in the gut can influence your mood. He identified *Bifidobacterium*, which is a bacterium that seems to have an anti-anxiety effect. Most probiotics are not psychobiotics, but *Bifidobacterium* is a probiotic that is a psychobiotic too. Professor Dinan later moved to Cork, where he was a principal investigator in the APC Microbiome Institute at UCC. We now know that gut microbiota, which are the community of microbiota living in our gut, are part of our stress system. Now we know that when the gut microbiome is altered our capacity to deal with stress is altered too. The brain–gut connection is like two communities living together in one house, needing each other to survive, but largely ignoring each other. Researchers continue to reveal connections between gut health and other diseases, both mental and physical. For example, there is now evidence the microbiome of IBS patients is altered. When a person has an unhealthy microbiome they are not as well equipped to deal with stress as they usually would be.

If you've ever had an upset stomach when you're stressed, or butterflies when you're nervous, you will already know about the way the brain and gut speak to each other. They are also physically connected by the vagus nerve and by chemicals called neurotransmitters.

The nerve cells in the intestinal wall are identical to those in the brain; they also use the same neurotransmitters to communicate. This is sometimes why we feel our gut is talking to us. Scientists now call this the abdominal brain: the intestine and brain are in permanent dialogue via the brain–gut axis, nerve pathways, metabolic products and hormones. We have 100 million nerve cells in the digestive tract. The telecommunication service between the brain and the gut is managed primarily by the tenth cranial nerve, the vagus nerve, which controls the internal organs and their function. Microbes in the gut can signal through the vagus nerve, which is a long meandering nerve that circles between the brain, gut and internal organs. *Lactobacilli* produce GABA (gamma-aminobutyric acid), which is a key transmitter that can have a tranquilising effect to reduce anxiety.

Neurotransmitters are usually found in the brain and run your feelings and emotions. Serotonin is the neurotransmitter that contributes to happiness. These neurotransmitters are also produced in your gut by the trillions of microbes that live there. A lot of serotonin is produced in the gut.

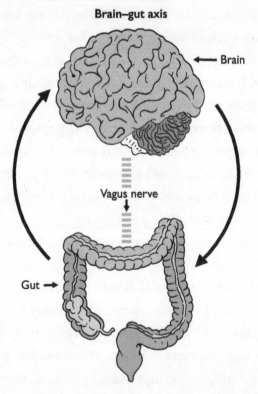

Brain–gut axis

More than 20 hormones are produced in the intestine. New studies show that our intestinal flora use enzymes to regulate our oestrogen levels. It is therefore assumed that poor gut health not only increases the risk of hormonally influenced disease but also influences hormone balance.

Much of our immune system is also affected by what happens in the gut and research into inflammatory bowel disease, ulcerative colitis and Crohn's disease has shown how the immune system is compromised when the bowel and gut aren't working optimally.

Inside everyone is a complex mix of trillions of microorganisms. Bacteria, viruses, fungi and other tiny life forms make up what we now call the microbiome and it plays a fundamental role in metabolic, nutritional and immune system functions in the body.

The intestinal flora get out of sync through stress, excessive work, jet lag, some medications, irregular food intake and a diet lacking in sufficient nutrition and fibre. A significant loss of bacteria in the gut, as can happen after a course of antibiotics, can cause an undersupply or oversupply of oestrogen. A microbiome that changes can also damage the blood vessels. We have long known that blood vessels grow stiffer with age. Research has now shown that in old age intestinal bacteria produce molecules which promote atherosclerosis (when arteries harden and become narrow).

Your microbiome make-up can be changed by things like antibiotic use, diet, probiotics and a procedure called a faecal microbial transplant, where a stool from a healthy person is transplanted via colonoscopy to a person suffering from a very specific type of colitis.

There are several diseases that are now thought to be influenced by what goes on in your gut microbiome. These include cancer, autoimmune disorders such as multiple sclerosis and autism spectrum disorder. The two important positive influences are a diverse diet with plenty of fruit and vegetables and good aerobic exercise.

Your unique microbiome

Gut microbiota are unique to each individual, and their composition is influenced by various factors, some of which we can control and others we cannot. People can support the balance of their gut microbiome by making healthy lifestyle choices such as the food they eat and how much exercise they get. In healthy bodies, the gut microbiota ferment non-digestible food components, mainly dietary fibre, to produce short-chain fatty acids that are important for maintaining a healthy colon.

Good sources of dietary fibre are whole grains (porridge for breakfast is a great option), vegetables with every meal, beans or legumes instead of meat, whole pieces of fruit for snacks, and nuts and seeds. As well as adding to your healthy microbiome, dietary fibre helps to relieve constipation, reduces the risks of cardiovascular diseases, Type 2 diabetes and certain cancers, helps with weight management, and improves oral and mental health.

Lymphoid tissues are organised structures that support immune responses. The gut-associated lymphoid tissue is highly specialised and is the main constituent of mucosal lymphoid tissue, representing 70% of the entire immune system. When the microbiome becomes imbalanced, which is known as dysbiosis, it can cause an increase in potentially harmful microbes, loss of microbial diversity and loss of beneficial microbes. Dysbiosis can be caused by antibiotics, gastritis, stress and lack of sleep.

You see, so much of our health comes back to stress and rest. Rest really is the most important gift that you can give yourself.

Small intestinal bacterial overgrowth (SIBO)

This is the overgrowth of normal gut bacteria in your small intestine and is the cause of 80% of cases of IBS. It also worsens perimenopause symptoms by impairing oestrogen removal from the body. It can worsen autoimmune thyroid disease too and it switches on the inflammatory system by activating mast cells.

The symptoms are abdominal bloating shortly after eating, nausea, pain and constipation. Its diagnosis is confirmed by a breath test. Treatment involves antibiotics and consulting with a dietitian who will instruct you about an appropriate diet such as the FODMAP diet mentioned in the previous chapter.

Probiotics and prebiotics

You may have had friends or family telling you to take acidophilus after a course of antibiotics to help with things like thrush. Well, they were right. Acidophilus is a probiotic and can help return the gut to a healthy state after dysbiosis.

Probiotics have many great benefits for your gut and microbiome and are found in lots of food sources like yoghurt, kefir, sauerkraut, pickles and even sourdough bread. Look out for the word 'live' to show that the food contains beneficial cultures. You can also find some great live probiotics in supplements (you often have to keep these in the fridge). Professor Dinan states that to have a good microbiome we should be taking in a lot of prebiotic fibre that acts as food for the psychobiotics.

Prebiotics are slightly different in that they are types of fibre that stimulate the growth of healthy bacteria. So where probiotics are replacing something, prebiotics are encouraging them to grow in the first place. You'll find them in bananas, artichokes, oats and apples among other things.

If you have a good, healthy, balanced diet, you'll already be packing in the prebiotics.

The microbiome and the menstrual cycle

A third of women experience cyclical changes in gut function and bowel habits associated with their menstrual function. The reason for this is most likely that hormones control muscles, including the bowel muscle. If there is a fluctuation of the FSH/ LH ratio causing menstrual irregularity, then the circadian rhythm of the bowel function will be affected. I liken this to the disruption of a conveyor belt where when one thing is disrupted there is a knock-on effect.

Hydration

Being well hydrated is very important for your overall health but how much you drink can have an impact on your hormones that you might not know about. We all need 2 litres of water a day but I always tell patients to try to drink some of it first thing in the morning because that helps with the bowel. You can have a glass the minute you get out of bed, then another glass with your breakfast, and one at 11 a.m. and another one at lunch, but don't have one after 7 p.m. Everything you have after this time is going to end up waking you in the middle of the night and disrupting your sleep, which you now know is vital for recharging your whole hormone system. That's the worst thing and I always tell patients not to drink anything after 7 p.m.

Hydration is vital because all your organs need it. We need it for the kidneys and skin. The blood needs a certain amount of hydration as well and the bowel needs it to work properly. But there is a 'but' here. Your pituitary gland controls the whole water system. There is a hormone in the posterior part of the pituitary gland called ADH or anti-diuretic hormone, which works on the kidneys to absorb water. If you drink too much water, you stop the function of ADH, and you can end up passing an unregulated amount of urine and will be constantly thirsty as well as a result. You're actually dehydrating yourself by drinking too much.

Again, I keep saying this, but it's about moderation and getting the balance right as opposed to extremes. Extremes of anything aren't good.

Stress and your metabolism

We know that too much stress is a bad thing but what happens to your metabolism when you experience ongoing stress?

Cortisol is the stress hormone and is produced naturally in your adrenal glands. It is released into your bloodstream when you're stressed and enables your body to react and go into fight or flight mode, pausing normal bodily functions while it deals with the danger and slowing your metabolism. This is all good and exactly what it should do in times of danger. But if you have very heightened cortisol, it's going to affect your immune system, it's going to increase your metabolic rate, and it's going to increase the oxidative stress in your body. That means that you have more free radicals breaking down cells. We know that that can cause heart disease and cancer, and it affects the immune system. With high cortisol everything functions the way it shouldn't, so you've got high oxidative stress, your immune system won't work well, and it will affect the arteries.

Raised levels of cortisol also create a boost of energy in your body, and this can increase your appetite and cause cravings for sweet, fatty, salty and carbohydrate-heavy foods. The combination of those cravings and your metabolism slowing can lead to fatigue, weight gain, depression, Type 2 diabetes and a poorly functioning immune system.

It can also impact fertility because when you have sustained levels of stress you get high levels of infertility. A woman came to me who had spent five years trying to get pregnant. She had come to see me first when she was devastated about her infertility. When I checked her hormones they were fine except for a raised prolactin level. I told her what I tell everyone, which is to try to control the stress in her life, eat as healthily as she could and rest, rest, rest. I know it can be frustrating to be told to relax and stop thinking about getting pregnant when it's something that you want so much but when the prolactin levels go up it inhibits ovulation and it is a direct result of stress.

When she came back to see me she was pregnant. She told me that she had stopped concentrating on conceiving, completely relaxed, did reflexology, ate healthfully and cut out sugar from her diet.

Ketogenic diets

Well, this will be a short section because I don't believe in them. A ketogenic diet is a high-fat and very low-carbohydrate diet that is similar to an Atkins diet. I am often told about special diets that cure this and that disease but I must work from the science. I have been seeing patients for 30 years and I have always said that the best diet is the simple healthy one. You cannot maintain a very restrictive, limited diet in the long term, and nor should you – it's no way to live. What we need are three meals a day with plenty of vegetables, lots of colour on the plate, and two small snacks.

Don't become an apple

As we age a lot of us tend to put weight on around our middle and that is not good for us. Abdominal fat – which is what causes the apple shape – is more insidious than fat that settles on our hips, bum or thighs. Abdominal fat has been linked to diabetes, heart disease and other metabolic abnormalities. Just because you're what is considered a healthy weight doesn't mean you're healthy. The scales may say you're fine but if you're carrying your weight around your middle you need to look at your diet and exercise. The risk increases for men when their waist measures more than 40 inches and for women at 35 inches.

The perfect diet

The perfect diet consists of fresh and organic meat, fish, eggs, fruit, vegetables, nuts and seeds. We should try to avoid processed food as much as possible. I know that it's very hard to have the perfect diet. We're all busy and trying our best to cook and eat healthy meals, but if you want to give your health the best chance, try to have the following foods in your diet.

Greek yoghurt

Studies suggest that we should eat good-quality Greek yoghurt every day and avoid the low-fat version that is full of sweeteners and sugar.

Chia seeds

Chia seeds contain more omega-3 fatty acids than salmon, more fibre than flax seed and a lot of antioxidants and minerals including phosphorus, manganese, calcium, potassium and sodium.

Eggs

An egg a day is within normal limits but do not exceed this amount because eggs contain cholesterol. If you want to have a two-egg omelette today, then avoid eggs tomorrow. Eggs are a great source of protein and help you stay fuller for longer. Most of the nutrients are found in the yolk, including vitamin B12, which helps the body metabolise fat, so don't be tempted to have an egg white omelette.

Green tea

Countless studies have shown that green tea helps to speed up metabolism and increases fat burning. It contains a compound called catechin which boosts energy expenditure, increases the release of fat from the cells and speeds up the liver's ability to burn fat. It is especially effective after meals so have a cup after your breakfast and lunch but not after dinner as it contains caffeine and may disrupt your sleep if you drink it too late in the day.

Green vegetables

These are filled with nutrients and have great health benefits. Kale has powerful antioxidant properties and asparagus is loaded with nutrients and antioxidants. Spinach is rich in Vitamin C and contains high levels of magnesium. It is also a great source of iron.

Avocados and oily fish

Avocados are a rich source of monounsaturated fat. Studies show that the healthy fat in avocado helps to absorb nutrients from solid ingredients up to five times more efficiently. The omega-3 fatty acids in oily fish like salmon, tuna and mackerel help to burn belly fat and speed up a slow metabolism. According to one Australian study, these sources of omega-3 stabilise the glucose-insulin response of the body which leads to a reduction of stomach fat.

Turkey

This contains an amino acid called leucine which helps prevent muscle mass loss during weight loss. Like all proteins, it helps keep you full and helps prevent muscle loss during weight loss plus it keeps your metabolism fired up. Include it in your evening meal a couple of times per week.

Berries

Berries contain anthocyanins, the plant chemicals which give them their bright colour and which help to burn abdominal fat. Studies show that stomach fat is more sensitive to the effects of anthocyanins than other types of body fat.

Coconut oil

This is one of the few oils that maintains its health benefits when heated. It also helps strengthen immunity and helps keep cholesterol levels healthy. When cooking on a medium heat you can use extra virgin olive oil but when cooking on a high heat use coconut oil.

Porridge and sweet potatoes

Porridge and other complex carbohydrate foods increase serotonin levels in the brain. Sweet potatoes contain more fibre and vitamins than regular white potatoes.

Nuts

Walnuts are high in fibre, antioxidants and unsaturated fatty acids, all of which help lower cholesterol and blood pressure.

Where and how you eat

We've talked about how what you eat impacts your hormonal health, but now let's talk about where and how you eat. You may remember growing up being told to sit at the table until you finished every last bite. In many households, there was no way you would even think about taking your dinner into another room or eating in front of the television, and yet that's how many of us eat now. A plate on our knees while watching the TV, a bite eaten in a hurry between meetings, a sandwich wolfed down in the car on the way to pick up or drop off. None of this is conducive to mindful eating or good digestion. You don't know if you're coming or going half the time, never mind if you're full or satisfied. Here's what I think you should try to do (also please note that I say 'try'; I don't want this to be another thing to feel guilty about, trying is good enough):

- If you're out at work, try to take a lunch break. Get away from your desk and your computer and remove yourself from where you've been sitting all morning. Sit outside (daylight is good for you), meet a friend or take a walk. Eat something you enjoy and that will give you energy for the rest of the day.

- Build in time to eat. We're all running from Billy to Jack, but meals are important and should be planned. Some days are harder than others but make the time to sit down for your lunch or your dinner, enjoy what you (or someone in your family) have made and chew your food and digest your meal.

- Keep snacking to a minimum. Picking away all day will mess with your blood sugars and you won't know when you're really hungry or full. Three meals a day and one or two small snacks are really all you need.

- Concentrate on the task at hand. Don't scroll on your phone or watch TV while eating. Your body won't know when it's full and if you are concentrating on a screen, you're likely to eat as many as 25% more calories!

- Chew your food – it's not a race and your body needs you to do it for proper digestion.

- You know about the division of protein, vegetables and carbohydrates that should be on your plate, but did you know you should also eat the protein and vegetables first?

You may not actually be hungry for that huge mound of mash on the side.

- Eat when you're hungry but don't wait until you're hangry (anger caused by hunger). Try to keep to a regular mealtime schedule. Equally, don't eat until you burst. It takes your brain about 20 minutes to catch up with your stomach and realise that it's full, so don't overeat.

CHAPTER EIGHT
Stress and Hormones

Quiz

1 In the last month, how often have you been upset because of something that happened unexpectedly?
2 In the last month, how often have you felt that you were unable to control the important things in your life?
3 In the last month, how often have you felt nervous and stressed?
4 In the last month, how often have you felt confident about your ability to handle your personal problems?
5 In the last month, how often have you felt that things were going your way?
6 In the last month, how often have you found that you could not cope with all the things that you had to do?

7 In the last month, how often have you been able to control irritations in your life?

8 In the last month, how often have you felt that you were on top of things?

9 In the last month, how often have you been angered because of things that happened that were outside of your control?

10 In the last month, how often have you felt difficulties were piling up so high that you could not overcome them?

These are the questions from the Perceived Stress Scale, which was first developed in 1983 and is still used today.

To score it you give each statement a rating from 0 to 4. For questions 1, 2, 3, 6, 9 and 10 score 0 for never, 1 for almost never, 2 for sometimes, 3 for fairly often and 4 for very often. For questions 4, 5, 7 and 8 mark them like this instead: never = 4, almost never = 3, sometimes = 2, fairly often = 1, very often = 0.

Add up your answers. Scores between 0 and 13 indicate low stress, between 14 and 26 moderate stress and between 27 and 40 high stress.

Managing our stress

Some stress is normal. You don't get through life without feeling it at some point. But for many people, modern life has created a situation where they live in a prolonged state of stress and that is not good for them. Lengthy periods of heightened stress are bad for our health. Stress can send your natural hormonal balance into a state of flux and can lead to insomnia, low libido, thyroid issues, fatigue, depression, stomach problems and anxiety.

Our bodies naturally create stress hormones like cortisol and adrenaline, and they help you react to situations that need quick reaction and attention. It could be a car accident or a huge presentation at work or nearly missing a flight, but whatever it is your heart will beat faster, your breath will quicken, and you'll feel your muscles tense up. This is called the fight or flight response and it's what gets you through the stressful situation.

If you've ever seen videos of people lifting cars to save someone or running for their lives and wondered how it's possible, that's the fight or flight reaction in action doing its job.

It's very necessary for some situations and it's built into our DNA from when we were literally running from beasts as we gathered our food. But in modern life, our bodies can react to less life-threatening situations with the same force. Traffic, pressure at work and problems at home can trigger the same response and cause chronic stress. This state of constant stress takes its toll on the body and research shows that chronic stress can contribute to high blood pressure, anxiety, depression, obesity, insomnia and addiction.

How does it work?

The stress response begins in the brain when you see or hear danger. This message is sent to the amygdala, an area of the brain that deals with emotional processing. That takes the information and when it perceives danger it immediately sends another message to the hypothalamus.

We know that the hypothalamus is a command centre sending messages all over the body. It communicates via the autonomic nervous system which controls involuntary functions like breathing, blood pressure and heartbeat. The autonomic nervous system is then broken up further into the sympathetic and parasympathetic nervous systems. They work in opposition to each other. Activation of the sympathetic nervous system leads to the fight or flight response, while a parasympathetic nervous system activation leads to a rest and digest response.

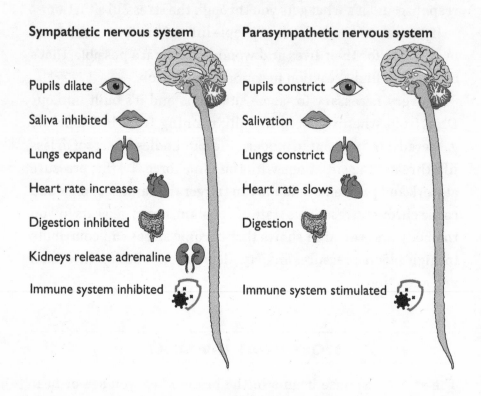

In fight or flight mode, the sympathetic nervous system changes how the body works and inhibits things it doesn't deem vital, like your digestive and immune systems. It increases pupil size, expands the lungs and releases adrenaline. These actions are supposed to help your body deal with an attack – you don't need to digest your food when you're in danger, but you definitely need to breathe better!

Stress and Hormones

The rest and digest response that the parasympathetic nervous system controls changes other functions to help it to recover. It's basically the opposite of what happens in fight or flight and includes decreasing heart rate and pupil size, restimulating the digestive and immune systems and contracting the lungs. This helps the body to have optimal rest and calms the body down after the perceived danger has passed.

Once the amygdala has sent its distress signal, the hypothalamus sends the sympathetic nervous system into action. Adrenaline, also known as epinephrine, is pumped into the bloodstream and causes physiological fight-or-flight changes. Of course, all of this happens so fast that you aren't even aware of it and it all starts before your brain has even told you what's happening.

As that first surge of adrenaline subsides, the hypothalamus fires up the HPA axis. This is the hypothalamus, the pituitary gland and the adrenal glands working together. The HPA axis relies on a series of hormonal signals to keep the sympathetic nervous system working. If the brain continues to see danger, the hypothalamus will release CRH (corticotropin-releasing hormone) which travels to the pituitary gland, triggering the release of ACTH (adrenocorticotropic hormone). This in turn makes its way to the adrenal glands, which then release cortisol and so the body stays on high alert.

What should happen next is that as cortisol levels fall, the parasympathetic nervous system should calm down the stress response. However, for many people that doesn't happen.

Chronic, low-level stress keeps the HPA axis activated by continually sending negative feedback, and it stays working away in the background for too long. After a while, this has an effect on the body and all the symptoms associated with chronic stress start to appear.

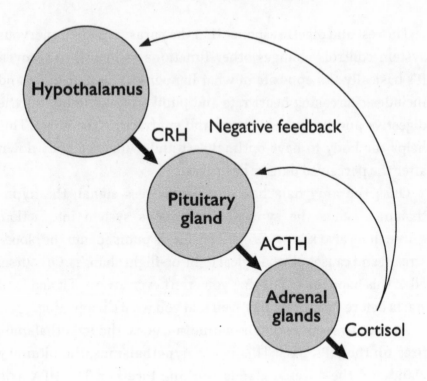

Living in this state can disrupt a lot of your body's processes and put you at risk of many health issues. Persistent adrenaline surges can damage arteries and blood vessels and leave you with high blood pressure, which raises your risk of heart attack and stroke. Cortisol increases appetite because you need to eat more for energy, but if you're not burning that off it can lead to the build-up of fat tissue and weight gain. Long-term activation of the HPA axis can also put you at risk of anxiety, depression, sleep issues, memory impairment, stomach problems and headaches.

Everyone reacts to stress differently. You might have two friends and one is so laid back they're almost horizontal while the other has huge reactions to seemingly small events. This is down to two things: genes and experience.

Some of our response to stress comes from our genetic make-up, while for others the reaction may be associated with traumatic events. People who experienced neglect or trauma as a child can be vulnerable to stress and the same is true for people who have been in major accidents or the victims of violent crime. Gardaí, paramedics, firefighters and hospital staff often also have different reactions to stress.

Where can you feel the effects of stress the most?

Muscle pain

When your body is in a state of stress your muscles tense up to protect it from injury. Chronic stress results in the muscles being in a constant state of tension due to hormonal imbalance. Muscles being tense for a prolonged period can result in stress-related conditions. Tension headaches and migraines are both linked to muscle hormonal imbalance and therefore muscle tension in the shoulders, neck and head. Muscle pain in the lower back has also been linked to stress, particularly stress at work.

Cardiovascular system

Chronic stress can mean an ongoing elevated heart rate, raised blood pressure and high levels of stress hormones such as adrenaline and cortisol, which can increase the risk of hypertension, heart attack or stroke. It can also result in inflammation in the circulatory system, especially of the coronary arteries, which can lead to a heart attack.

The risk of stress-related heart disease differs for women depending on whether they are premenopausal or postmenopausal. Normal levels of oestrogen help premenopausal women's blood vessels respond better during stress, while postmenopausal women lose this protection due to lower levels of oestrogen. HRT offers some protection against this but only up to 60 years of age.

Gastrointestinal system

We've already spoken about the brain–gut axis and stress can affect this communication. Stress is associated with changes in the bacteria that live in the gut, which can then impact mood.

The oesophagus

Stressed people often experience changes in their diet; they might eat more or less than usual and/or increase their use of alcohol or tobacco. All of this can result in heartburn or acid reflux. Stress can make people eat faster and swallow more air when eating, or make swallowing difficult, which increases burping, bloating and flatulence. Stress interferes with hormones and hormones control muscles (remember that the oesophagus is a muscular organ).

The stomach

If stress is severe enough it can cause vomiting, nausea and stomach pain. While stress doesn't cause stomach ulcers, it can make them worse.

The bowel

Anyone with a nervous stomach will know that stress can affect the bowel. Increased adrenaline increases the motility of the bowel. It can affect how quickly food moves through your system, which can cause diarrhoea or constipation. It particularly affects people who already have a chronic bowel condition like inflammatory bowel disease or IBS.

Female reproductive system

Stress can affect your menstrual cycle and can change the length of your cycle, causing painful or absent periods. Sexual desire can be impacted by chronic stress as fatigue and low mood reduce libido. It can also make PMS symptoms worse. Stress can have a big impact on a woman's ability to conceive as it increases prolactin levels and therefore inhibits ovulation. While menopause can be a stressor itself, chronic stress can make the physical symptoms of menopause worse – a vicious circle.

What can you do to combat stress?

It's easy to say relax, but it's not as easy to do. There is a practice called the relaxation response where you train your body to relax. It involves deep abdominal breathing, visualisation and physical practices such as yoga and tai chi. The relaxation response was first described by a Harvard Medical School professor called Herbert Benson more than 40 years ago. He found that it was helpful in the treatment of stress-related disorders.

Physical activity is recommended to calm the build-up of stress. Something like a brisk walk after a period of stress will help to deepen breathing and relax muscle tension. Yoga and tai chi combine movement with focused breathing, which can help bring a feeling of calm too. Removing yourself from the stressor and concentrating on something that uses the whole body can help to calm that HPA axis.

Having social support is also proven to help with chronic stress. 'Don't suffer in silence' is something we hear a lot, but it has a basis in truth. Having family, friends and colleagues in whom you can confide has been shown to increase longevity. A social circle and having the protection of emotional support at difficult times is a good buffer from chronic stress.

Burnout and stress go hand in hand and if you feel things are getting on top of you, step back and take a look at your life. Do you need to pull back on something for a while? Are you stretching yourself so you can include exercise in your routine or are you working longer and longer hours because your desk is in your spare room? Small changes can make a big difference and if you need to cut something out to ease the pressure on yourself you should. Your long-term health will thank you for it.

Lifestyle changes to deal with stress

- Have hobbies.
- Make time for family and friends.
- Eat a healthy diet and get exercise.
- Make sleep a priority – rest is important.
- Try to have a sense of humour and laugh at life.
- Volunteer.
- Practise yoga or meditation.
- Get counselling to learn how to cope with stress.
- Speak to a professional if you feel you can't manage.
- Don't rely on alcohol, drugs, tobacco or food to make you feel better.

Remember that we have lived through one of the most stressful events that this generation will ever see. The global Covid-19 pandemic not only changed our lives for two years, but it has changed work patterns and society for ever.

That is a lot to contend with and we all have felt stressed at some point or other. It's not stress itself that is bad – sometimes you can't avoid it – it's how we deal with it and how frequently we let it affect us that is the issue. Find coping mechanisms that work for you.

That could be time alone to switch off, a day laughing with friends or a powerful workout – whatever it is, make it a priority. Life can be hard, but it's harder when we're overstressed and overtired. I see it all the time in my clinics and people often don't even realise that they're living with chronic stress as it's been part of their lives for so long.

Reduce coffee

Irish people often reach for the kettle at times of stress but that hit of caffeine may not be doing you any good. If you're able to have one cup in the morning that's fine, but if you're on four or five cups a day, the hit of energy isn't worth it. You can end up in an insomnia-caffeine-insomnia loop that is hard to escape from and does nothing for your stress levels. If you find yourself stressed and in perimenopause, it's worth giving up coffee altogether and seeing what that does for your mood and symptoms. Caffeine can be a contributory factor in hot flushes.

CHAPTER NINE

Sleep and Hormones

You simply can't overestimate the importance of rest in your life. It is the one thing we can all do that will make a difference. But you'll tell me, and believe me when I say I hear this all the time, 'I can't', 'I work late', 'I only get to the housework after the children go to bed', 'the children don't sleep', 'I've to get up early to go to my 6 a.m. exercise class' or 'I've emails to answer after dinner'. To all that I simply say, no. You're doing too much, and you'll make yourself sick. It's as simple as that.

If you need to keep working when you get home, there's a disconnect at work. If you only get to the housework in the evening, get a cleaner if you can (I will assume that if you have a partner or children they are already helping, because if they're not, we have a whole other problem to deal with).

If you're caring for elderly relations who keep you up at night, ask other family members if they can step in to help share the burden. If your children don't sleep and you're the one up with them, share that burden so you're not the only one exhausted. If you're getting up at 6 a.m. to exercise and you're exhausted, stop it. Sleep trumps exercise.

I have an answer for everything, and isn't that annoying? Well, it's easy for her, you might say, but I have a house, a job and children too. I am a widowed mother of three, working full time, and I make sure to prioritise rest. It's not always easy but I know how important it is and you should too.

One of the main things doctors are asked for is a tonic for tiredness. People come and say, 'I'm exhausted all the time, I'm tired in the morning, I need my bloods checked and something to take.' The first thing I will always do is ask them about their schedules, their evenings and their sleep. It is incredible the number of people who come to see me and can tell me exactly how little sleep they're getting and what poor quality it is because their smartwatch is tracking it. They have all the facts right there on their wrist and yet they're doing nothing about it.

Do you know what I prescribe to these patients? It's an absolute miracle cure – rest and Vitamin Sleep.

What your body does while you sleep

Sleep gives your body and mind time to rest and reset. Your mother might have told you that you'd feel better after a good night's sleep, and she was right. Everything always seems much worse when you're tired and stressed and there's a reason that you can deal with life better after some rest.

Repair

Several different hormones are released while you sleep, all with different jobs to do. Melatonin is released by the pineal gland, and this controls your sleep patterns. Levels of melatonin increase at night time and it helps to send you to sleep. While you're asleep, growth hormone is released by the pituitary gland and helps your body to grow and to repair.

Immune boost

The reason you need lots of sleep when you're sick is that the body uses this time to heal. While you're asleep, your immune system releases cytokines. These are small proteins that work to help you fight infection and inflammation. Sleep helps your body function properly.

Making memories

One part of your body that's still busy when you're sleeping is the brain. It uses this time to process everything that happened during the day. Think of it like a big filing system. Your brain sorts out all the information it's gathered during the day and files it away for the future. This is how it stores long-term memories.

Sympathetic sleep

We've already talked about stress, and sleep is an important factor in recovering from fight or flight mode. Sleep gives your sympathetic nervous system a chance to slow down and relax. It has been proven that when we're sleep-deprived our sympathetic nervous system activity increases and our blood pressure rises, which we know can cause chronic stress.

Ready for the day

Alongside melatonin, cortisol levels drop as you sleep and then slowly rise again to wake you up. They also switch on your appetite so you're ready to fuel up for the day ahead.

Clever work

Your body does lots of really smart things that you don't ever really know about! While you sleep your body releases ADH, the anti-diuretic hormone. That's why, even though you may have to pee several times a day, you can go eight hours without having to use the bathroom. So clever!

Sleep and women

According to the National Sleep Foundation in the US, the risk of suffering from insomnia is 40% higher for women than it is for men. Some of that has to do with hormones but some of it has to do with the extra workload women tend to take on: the emotional labour of running a house and family. If we're already at a disadvantage for sleep due to our hormonal make-up, it should make sense that everything involved in keeping the house and family going should be shared equally. Right?

The hormonal impact on a woman's sleep starts early. When puberty starts and girls begin to menstruate it triggers a 40-year cycle of hormonal fluctuations that can impact sleep. Before this, there is no difference in sleep levels for boys and girls. Puberty changes that.

The hormone level that affects sleep for women is progesterone. In the days before your period, progesterone levels rise, getting your body ready for a potential period. When there is no implantation those levels drop dramatically, which is why some women can find it hard to get good-quality sleep in the days before and during their period. When bleeding stops, those progesterone levels rise again and sleep becomes easier.

In polycystic ovary syndrome (PCOS), irregular periods and cycles mean lower levels of progesterone, which means that women with PCOS often have poor-quality sleep.

Pregnant women often complain about 'pregnancy insomnia' and it's a very real thing. Hormones race through your body to support your growing baby and things can get a bit rough. In the first three months, progesterone levels rise to help keep the uterus relaxed and the immune system working; oestrogen also rises dramatically at this time. Pregnant women often talk about being tired all day and awake all night and it's no wonder with this cocktail of hormones racing around.

By the third trimester, hormone levels will have levelled out but by then other factors like restless legs, the baby's position on your bladder and breathing difficulties can make it hard to get enough sleep. Keeping your head elevated, lots of pillows and relaxation techniques can help.

Sleep and the menopause

You're not done with sleep problems when you get to your menopause years, though. In perimenopause, hormone levels start messing with sleep once again. As your cycle changes and slows, your hormones begin to fluctuate and you start to get symptoms like hot flushes, night sweats and restless legs, which can all impact your sleep. As well as these physical symptoms, lower levels of progesterone can also cause irritability in some women and make them less able to relax. HRT and a replacement of the lost oestrogen can help women to sleep better. Sleeping issues are considered to be one of the main symptoms of perimenopause and menopause. Between 40% and 60% of women report symptoms of sleeplessness and insomnia during this time.

Urinary problems also pose an issue for sleep for women in perimenopause and menopause. Frequent urination at night and other issues related to an overactive bladder impact sleep and women are twice as likely as men to experience urinary incontinence. Low levels of oestrogen can weaken the bladder and urethra.

While it's common for men to snore and suffer from sleep apnoea women are somewhat protected from it by progesterone and oestrogen, but as those levels fall in perimenopause and menopause that benefit is lost. Older women are just as prone to sleep apnoea as men and it really impacts sleep. It has also been seen that women in menopause spend less time in REM sleep and they feel less rested when they wake.

REM sleep

When you sleep, your brain moves through five different stages. One of these is REM or rapid eye movement sleep. You enter the REM stage about 90 minutes after falling asleep and it repeats as you move through your sleep cycles. Most of your dreams happen when you're in REM sleep and it is thought to play a part in learning, memory and mood. REM accounts for about 50% of children's sleep and about 25% of adults' sleep. Different phases of REM last for different lengths of time. The first lasts just 10 minutes while the final one can last for up to an hour, which is why you often remember the dreams you have just before you wake up. Having alcohol affects the amount of REM sleep you have, which is why you tend to feel less well rested after you've been drinking.

Sleep debt

You might have heard of the term sleep debt; it's also called sleep deficit and is the difference between the amount of sleep you need and the amount of sleep you get. Everyone needs a different amount of sleep but if you generally need eight hours' sleep to work at your optimal level and you only get six hours, you have two hours of sleep debt. Sleep debt is also cumulative so if you lose an hour a night by going to bed later or being woken by children that debt builds up quite fast.

People with very young children and those working shift hours usually have the highest level of sleep debt. This debt does have consequences. As well as feeling tired generally, it can impact work and driving and increase the risk of diabetes, heart disease, high blood pressure and stroke. It also interferes with your immune system and metabolism. If you have a period of prolonged sleep deprivation, it can also affect your cognitive functions.

Women are more likely than men to build up sleep debt. Not only do women and men deal with a lack of sleep differently but women also usually shoulder the burden of night feeds for small children, which builds up that debt very quickly.

So what can you do to clear the debt? First and foremost, get more sleep. If your sleep debt is child-related, go to bed earlier and share the night-time wakes with your partner. Take naps; naps have been shown to help cognitive function. Try not to worry about child-related sleep debt – they all learn how to sleep eventually. If you're staying up late to scroll on your device and are having difficulty getting to sleep, cut screen time for at least an hour before bedtime.

The hormones related to sleep

There are several hormones that are related to sleep and they're all quite important. Getting quality sleep is important to keep them regulated and working properly. They include cortisol, oestrogen and progesterone, the hunger hormones (insulin, leptin and ghrelin), melatonin, thyroid hormones and the growth hormones.

Almost every hormone in your body is released in response to the sleep–wake cycle. It's a carefully balanced system that can easily become chaotic if those circadian rhythms are out of sync.

Melatonin

There has been a lot of discussion around melatonin in recent years and many people now take it as a supplement to help them get to sleep; you can get it on prescription from your GP. It's a hormone produced by the pineal gland that regulates your circadian rhythm so that you fall asleep, and crucially, stay asleep. Your circadian rhythm is influenced by the sun, which is why it's important to get outside and get daylight during the day, especially if you work in a place lit by artificial light. Melatonin levels drop during the day so that you stay awake and rise again as you approach bedtime. But those levels can be affected by the blue light produced by your electronic devices, which is why it's crucial to put them down at least an hour before you go to sleep.

Cortisol

Cortisol helps to regulate other hormones in the body and sleep regulates the amount of cortisol that the adrenal glands produce. Cortisol helps you to wake and then it tells all your other hormones, like your thyroid and oestrogen, to get to work.

If you don't sleep well, cortisol can interfere with the delicate balance of oestrogen and progesterone in your body. It can also cause your thyroid to slow down, which in turn affects your metabolism.

Hunger hormones

Have you ever noticed that you get really hungry when you're tired? That's because a lack of sleep affects the levels of hunger hormones in the body. This can impact appetite and can potentially lead to weight gain. Poor sleep impacts leptin, ghrelin and insulin and they are the hormones that are responsible for fullness, hunger, fat storage and blood sugar. Even just one night of poor sleep can interfere with insulin levels and over time that can become an issue.

Growth hormone

HGH or human growth hormone is really important for a number of reasons, but its main job is to maintain, build and repair the brain and other organs. If you've been injured, this is the hormone that is sent to help you to heal and it also helps to burn fat, build muscle and boost your metabolism. When you don't get enough sleep, the production of HGH is impacted. It is also said to help the appearance of skin – so you're literally getting your beauty sleep!

What does too little sleep do to your hormones?

Everyone's need for sleep is different. Some people do really well on six or seven hours while others definitely need the full eight or even nine hours of sleep. The right amount of sleep for you is the amount that allows you to wake refreshed and operate to your full potential each day. It is not the amount that you can just about get by on. That will not do at all. Not only will you end up completely burned out, but you won't get anything done well and you'll be grouchy, short-tempered and often upset. Remember that too little sleep impacts your immune system, and we know, having been through a global pandemic, that your immune system is something to be treasured, nurtured and minded.

It's very important to get a good night's sleep as regularly as you can. If you only sleep for five hours a night for a full week, you'll end up with a sleep debt that you can't catch up on in just one weekend – unless you can take to your bed for a full 24 hours and who among us can do that?

Not only do you need to have enough hours, but you also need to have good quality sleep that is both long enough and deep enough to allow for REM sleep. That's what will refresh and reset you.

Poor-quality sleep or just not enough sleep at all upsets the delicate hormone balance in your body and you know now that as soon as that is disrupted a lot can go wrong.

Sleep and your health

At this stage, you will know how important I consider rest to be to your overall health and well-being. I am genuinely concerned that modern life is putting our health at risk. We are not allowing ourselves the time to sleep properly or to rest and recuperate.

I love holidays with my family, and I see them as a crucial part of my well-being. They give me a chance to step away from daily life and enjoy myself at a slow and restful pace. If you're not taking your time off or not even allowing yourself some downtime at the weekends to sit and do very little, you're doing yourself and your health a massive disservice.

There's nothing worse than a busy fool and we're all allowing busyness to creep into our lives at a completely unsustainable rate. If you run on empty you won't eat well, you'll be stressed, exhausted and will become unwell. Get a good night's sleep, take time off work and have a lovely snooze on the sofa after Sunday dinner. You deserve it.

Babies and young children

There are no doubt going to be mothers of young children reading this who are terrified at what the lack of sleep they're currently experiencing is doing to their bodies. There are always going to be times in your life when sleep is harder to come by than others and I accept and appreciate that. But there is still a lot you can do. You might think I should have said 'parents' there instead of mothers, but it is my experience that still in this day and age it is the woman on maternity leave who will be up four or five times a night with a child. I don't think that's good enough.

Simply because a woman looking after children is not leaving the house to go to an office every day does not mean that she is not working. Anyone who has looked after a small child all day knows that it definitely is work! Many women are expected to do this important job while surviving on cat naps for months at a time. Talk about burning out.

Breastfeeding mothers often experience this the most. I am a huge advocate of breastfeeding but not at the expense of the mother's health. A sick and exhausted mother is good for no one. If it is possible, I would like breastfeeding mums to pump and bottle feed one night a week so that they can get at least one full night's sleep. There must be time for naps too. The burden must be shared; there must be equality in the parental relationship so that women are not so exhausted they lose all sight of themselves.

Remember that being a new parent is an exhausting time and that, although it may feel like it when you're in the thick of it, it doesn't last for ever – wait until you have teens who won't get out of bed at all!

There is time to catch up on sleep and the body is amazing, it is doing a lot to protect new mothers in the background. Just make sure to rest when you can and speak to your family about how tired you are; as soon as you vocalise it, someone will step in to help. Don't try to muddle through – no one ever thanks a martyr.

Your brain needs sleep

When you sleep your brain activity falls into two categories – four stages of non-REM sleep and then a REM stage.

In stage one, your brain starts to produce alpha-theta waves as you fall asleep. These slow brainwaves help you to relax deeply and reduce your eye movements for a very light sleep stage that lasts around seven minutes. Then in stage two those brainwaves increase quickly and are known as sleep spindles. If you like to nap, this is the stage where you should wake up. A 10–20-minute nap will stop you from feeling groggy. After that point, your brain starts to produce delta waves, which are very slow waves that are very important. These are stages three and four and this slow-wave sleep is vital for brain functions like cognitive memory processing and remembering things like names and faces.

The final phase is REM sleep, which completes each 90-minute sleep cycle. REM sleep is where you dream and it's an important time for advanced learning, creativity and emotion, and long-term memory.

All these functions are why a bad night's sleep takes its toll. If you don't sleep well regularly, it can lead to attention and cognition problems, bad moods, anxiety and long-term insomnia.

Sleep hygiene

You might think that the term sleep hygiene is a bit new age, but it is vital to making sure we get enough good rest. Our lives are so intertwined with technology now and that is harming our sleep. Whether it's staying up too late binge-watching something on the television or lying in bed at night scrolling through our phones, it's having a negative impact. Technology can make it harder to fall asleep, but it can also make it more difficult to stay asleep; you may be having little micro-awakenings that you don't even realise are happening but mean that you're not getting good-quality rest. Here are some key steps for good sleep hygiene:

Routine

Try to go to bed at the same time every night. There will, of course, be nights where this isn't possible, but as often as you can stick to a routine. That includes the weekends!

Caffeine

Don't drink caffeine in the afternoon. You may think it's not affecting you, but it most probably is. Have a cup or two before midday and then switch to water or caffeine-free herbal teas.

Alcohol

A couple of drinks in the evening might help you nod off, but it won't help you to stay asleep. Alcohol is one of the biggest disruptors of sleep, so try to limit your intake.

Technology

These days technology is probably the number one sleep disruptor. The blue light that comes from our devices plays havoc with our circadian rhythm and watching a screen close to bedtime can make it difficult to fall asleep. You should put your phone, tablet and laptop down at least one hour before bedtime to give your body a chance to settle down and switch off. If you wake up during the night, resist the urge to look at your phone, as it will make nodding off again really hard. Keeping your phone in another room altogether and investing in an old-school alarm clock can be a really helpful way of breaking your night-time phone habit.

Night shift workers

Another group of people who are negatively affected by a lack of sleep are night shift workers. They come home after work and should go straight to bed, but many have guilt associated with day sleep and it has been shown that they often sleep half the number of hours as everyone else. I understand the world is carrying on, things are busy, and you feel you're wasting time while you're asleep. It's hard to prioritise rest but you must. I've met people who work night shifts who use the daytime to schedule house maintenance and hairdressing appointments and do all the school dropoffs and pickups. That is unsustainable. Someone who works late shifts or all-night shifts is as entitled to the same eight hours of sleep as everyone else. We must change the narrative.

It can be hard to sleep when the world is awake but here are some things you can do to make it easier on yourself.

Your circadian rhythm

You will be tired finishing work but as soon as you step out into daylight your body clock will tell you that it's the morning and will try hard to wake you up. If possible, park underground and wear good UV-filtering sunglasses all the way home (yes, even on an overcast day) – you need to trick your body into thinking it's the end of the day, not the start.

No caffeine at work. I mean it!

This is very hard, I know, as a cup of tea or coffee when you're exhausted at work is a great pick-me-up, but it won't help your sleep in the long run. Try to get used to caffeine-free herbal teas or plain water if you can. It will be hard at first to wean yourself off caffeine, but it will do you and your rest the world of good in the long run.

Food to help you sleep

Think about what you're going to eat before you get into bed. Have something that is comforting, filling and easy to digest. Remember to make sure you're well hydrated. People are often worried that their sleep will be disturbed by the need to wake up to go to the bathroom but being dehydrated will disrupt your sleep too so neither is a good idea. Be clever about not drinking water too close to bedtime, though, as you will need to get up to empty your bladder and it will affect your sleep routine.

Invest in your bedroom

Do things that make it easier to sleep. Get blackout blinds and curtains; they're not just for children, they help daytime sleepers to fall asleep too. Get good-quality bedlinens that keep you comfortable and cosy in the winter and cool in the summer. If you live in a busy place, invest in earplugs. Normal daytime sounds can be disruptive to sleep.

Let go of that guilt

This really is the most important thing. You deserve your rest so make sure you get it.

Tired all the time

If you change your habits and start to get enough good-quality sleep but you are still tired, your doctor will assess you for other causes of your exhaustion. It might be that prolonged time without sleep when you were burning the candle at both ends left you with a hormonal imbalance that needs to be sorted out, but there can be other causes too. Tiredness, even when you're sleeping well, can be caused by a number of things including:

- Type 1 or Type 2 diabetes
- Hyperthyroidism and hypothyroidism
- Undiagnosed infections
- Conditions like inflammatory bowel disease or Crohn's disease
- Conditions linked to your diet, such as low levels of vitamin B12
- Anxiety and depression

When to speak to a professional

If you're trying hard to improve your sleep and it's just not working for you, you should always speak to your doctor. You may have a sleep disorder or need some help getting your sleep back on track. As well as the lifestyle changes we've discussed here, there are other things you can do such as therapies for insomnia, relaxation therapies and prescription medications, though these are not long-term solutions and should be taken for the shortest amount of time possible.

CHAPTER TEN
Self-Esteem

'It took me a long time to develop my voice and now that I have it, I am not going to be silent.' – Madeleine Albright

We've come to the end of our journey into hormonal health but there's one more chapter and it's one that I feel is the key to everything we've learned so far.

A lot of the work I do now is about encouraging empowerment in the women I speak to. I am an endocrinologist and a medical doctor (not a psychologist), but in my experience, a lot of women I see have low self-esteem. While women have become more empowered in the last few years, we still need to see a lot more changes. Dr Tony Humphreys, a well-known Irish psychologist, has said that when we work too hard we often do it to become visible because we do not feel visible to ourselves. This is an extremely sad thought. It must change.

You may not even recognise it in yourself until I start to ask you questions about your home or work life, your tiredness and your health. Hormonal health is about balance, but how much of your life is balanced?

Busyness is something that society has decided to reward, and I don't know why. Fitting in exercise early in the morning before work, getting children ready for their day, going to work, coming home to make a meal for your family before you log back on to do yet more work, answer emails and sit in front of a screen until you drag yourself to bed is not balance.

Having it all is possible but only when you decide what 'it all' really is and when to ask for help. Whether you're single and trying to manage work, friendships and family responsibilities or you have a partner and a family and you're trying to be the world's best wife and mum, it's not okay to do all this without support.

But asking for help doesn't always come easily to Irish women. It's a generational dysfunction that we are allowing to continue and is a cycle that needs to be broken. We need to empower ourselves and the next generation to be equal. If there are two partners in a relationship, everything should be shared 50/50.

If you are a daughter with elderly parents and the care falls to you and not your brothers, you must ask why. If you're a mum and you're carrying the mental load of after-school activities, summer camps, Santa visits and playdates without support, things have to change.

All the caring for family, children, the elderly and the home has traditionally fallen on the shoulders of women and it's time to shake that up and say that it's no longer acceptable. The world is still built for a life that we have all outgrown, for a time when a man went out to work and a woman looked after everything else.

When both partners are working, that is no longer a viable setup. Even when one partner works outside the home and the other is at home with children, it's time to acknowledge that being a stay-at-home parent is an exhausting role. I would like to see equality in life.

Women have been socialised to be good, polite, people-pleasers. It is of course lovely to be polite and pleasant, but this should not come at the expense of our well-being and happiness. You should not come last on the list of people in your life who need to be happy. How can you expect everyone around you to be happy when you are miserable or utterly burned out?

You have read over and over again in this book how the key to hormonal health is rest and recuperation. We are allowing ourselves to become exhausted by life and accept that exhaustion as normal.

We learn by watching, and if the next generation sees us cleaning, cooking, working and running after everyone else before doing anything for ourselves, just as our mothers did, we are not breaking the cycle, we are perpetuating it.

Having it all is only possible when you are empowered.

Seven questions of self-esteem

- Do you feel tired?
- Do you put other people's needs ahead of your own?
- Do you feel obligated to do it all?
- Do you find it hard to say no?
- Are you self-critical?
- Do you feel time-poor?
- Do you feel resentful?

Think about your answers here and then think about what you would say to your friends or sisters or daughters if they spoke to you about feeling this way. You would certainly give them a pep talk, tell them that they must slow down, that they should ask for help, wouldn't you? Now think about how you speak to yourself and how you react to the answers you gave to the questions. We must all learn to speak to ourselves the way we speak to our friends, sisters and daughters. We must give ourselves the same advice and take it.

Self-esteem and Maslow's Hierarchy of Needs

Abraham Maslow was an American psychologist who is best known for his theories about human behaviour and human needs.

His Hierarchy of Needs shows the spectrum of human needs. Some are physiological and needed to survive and others are psychological. Maslow described the needs as fluid, with many needs being present in a person at the same time.

At the bottom of the pyramid are the basic or physiological needs, which are necessary for survival. These include food, sleep, water, excretion, warmth, sex and homeostasis (a state of balance in the body).

The next level is safety needs: security, order and stability. These are your health, your personal and financial stability, your employment and the stability of your family.

Self-Esteem

The third level is love and belonging needs and this is where you move into psychological needs. Once you have secured yourself and feel safe, you are ready to share yourself with others. Belonging refers to our need for relationships, feeling connected and being part of a group.

Now we get to esteem needs, which include self-worth, accomplishment and respect. Maslow divided these into two categories. First is esteem for yourself, citing elements like dignity, independence and achievement, and second comes the desire for respect from others, including status and prestige.

At the top of the pyramid is self-actualisation, which is when a person is working to achieve their full potential.

There are two other levels in the pyramid between esteem and self-actualisation that are not always shown. They are cognitive needs, which include knowledge, understanding, curiosity and the need for meaning; and aesthetic needs, which are an appreciation of beauty and balance.

Maslow said that the order of the needs isn't as rigid as the pyramid makes them look and they are different for each person. For some, the need for esteem outweighs the need for love, while for others the search for fulfilment might be more important than even the most basic needs.

What is interesting, however, is that Maslow included esteem as essential to human behaviour.

How do you empower yourself?

Eleanor Roosevelt once said that no one can make you feel inferior without your consent, and I believe that is so true. We must take an active role in empowering ourselves and a lot of that work starts with self-esteem. You must believe yourself to be as worthy as everyone else to become empowered.

How to empower yourself

- Stand up for yourself.
- Put the gaze on yourself (as the well-known Irish psychologist Dr Tony Humphreys always advises).
- Say NO to people and know your boundaries.
- Think positive, empowering thoughts. *The Power is Within You* is an excellent book by Louise Hay that I would recommend.
- Choose to be a warrior, not a victim.
- Take care of yourself.
- Only surround yourself with people who empower you and treat you as an equal.
- Empower others and give back.

CASE HISTORY: LOUISE

Louise was 45 when I first met her. She had tried for years to get pregnant and finally did when I settled her hormonal imbalance. She was elated to be pregnant after the long wait. Like a lot of women, she had suffered silently when she saw her sisters and friends getting pregnant and cried inwardly when people asked if she wanted to have children. Thankfully, most, though not all, people have now copped on and have stopped commenting on this very sensitive and private issue that a couple may be going through. It's very hurtful to be asked all the time when you're going through something so difficult.

Louise delivered a beautiful baby girl but I was shocked to get a hysterical phone call from her in the hospital. She had wanted to give her baby a double-barrelled surname so that both parents would be represented but she told me that her husband said he would not allow it.

Louise was an only child herself and wanted her family surname to continue. This was important to her. She had endured a lot to conceive this lovely baby girl and was hurt at her husband's lack of understanding.

I listened to her and then I said if in 30 years she got a call from her daughter to say her husband is not allowing her to give her surname to their child, what would she say to her? She responded by saying she 'would kill him', metaphorically speaking of course. I asked her why she would have that reaction for her daughter but not for herself. She realised that it was because she adored her new baby girl and would do anything for her, but she did not love herself as much.

Once she realised this she was empowered to act. She insisted on adding her surname to her husband's for their child and told him to get over his sulking and that she would not tolerate it any further. It was a major turning point in her life and a very positive one. It was also a very important defining point for her daughter who was now going to be growing up in a house where her mother was empowered and seeing herself as equal to her husband instead of a very different scenario. She was now an excellent role model and mentor for her daughter and her descendants and had started to break that dysfunctional intergenerational cycle.

If you place as much importance on yourself as you do on other people, you will start to see change. You will eat better, prioritise your rest, make time for your health and exercise and recognise a healthy work–life balance.

Here are some ways to lean into your own power and self-worth:

- **Know yourself well.** Take the time to figure out what you want from work and life. Only when you know that can you make plans to get there.
- **Set goals.** It can be easy to say 'Oh, I'll start that next month or when the kids are a bit older.' If you set both short- and long-term goals you are always working towards something and always achieving, even in little increments. This helps you feel focused and successful.

- **Challenge yourself.** It might be time to get out of your comfort zone and push yourself. You'll have new experiences and meet new people along the way.
- **Find your tribe.** Men have been great at networking for years and women should be doing the same thing. Find a network of support that empowers you and builds you up. It could be a professional organisation or a book club; just find the people who want you to succeed. If you are finding it hard to find that group, consider starting one yourself.
- **Build your confidence.** Some people say fake it till you make it, but I say you are what you believe. Being nervous is fine but don't let it take over. Try new things that help you feel more confident every day.

Empower others

Your empowerment is important but teaching the next generation to be empowered is vital. We must do everything we can to break the damaging intergenerational cycles in society. It can be as simple as empowering our children to find solutions to their problems or teaching both our sons and daughters to cook for themselves and do their own laundry, or it could be bigger than that, for example becoming a mentor to a young colleague or student. The best gift we can give our children is self-esteem.

We all want to help our children, nieces, nephews and young friends as much as we can but we're not helping them at all if we do it all for them. In order to help them grow into confident, able and empowered adults we must guide and advise and then step back and let them find their way.

CASE HISTORY: SINÉAD

In rural Irish life, there is often an imbalance in the roles we apply to men and women. I grew up in a farming family, so I have seen this first-hand.

When Sinéad came to see me she had difficult menopausal symptoms and severe fatigue. She was looking after her elderly father who had had a stroke and her mother who had Parkinson's disease. She was doing all this alone even though she had a brother who lived next door. He was farming and was deemed too busy to help.

Eighteen months after her first appointment, Sinéad came back to see me and broke down in the clinic. Both her parents had died in the year and a half since I had seen her last, which was terrible, but what was very upsetting was that they had left everything to her brother.

The most upsetting thing for her was their lack of respect for her and what she had done. This upset her far more than the financial element. She had worked night and day to look after them both. She was particularly angry with her mother. This is very common.

We see the mother as the nurturer, and we always blame the mother more even though both father and mother were responsible for her upset here. Now that they were gone, Sinéad could see the dysfunctional cycle she had been in and the lack of respect that her parents had shown her.

I have seen daughters left out of wills many times in my life. Families believe that daughters have husbands to look after them and that their sons are more deserving of the family home, farm or whatever they have to bequeath. It is something that can tear families apart and devastate daughters and it desperately needs to change. I hope that we are near the end of this terrible cycle in Irish family life and that the voices of empowered women will be heard.

I could only help Sinéad to get back on her feet hormonally, speak to her about her self-esteem and hope that she could move on from her hurt. I also referred her to a psychologist for help, which she found very beneficial. She came to me a few months later to say she was taking a case to reclaim her rightful inheritance to show her children that she saw herself as equal even if her parents did not. She was determined to break the dysfunctional cycle in her family.

Boundaries

A big part of empowerment is setting boundaries. Being able to say no is vital to protecting your well-being. Your time is as valuable as anybody else's and once you understand that you free up so much of the anxiety around saying no. Block off time for your own needs. Whether you do that physically in your diary or in your head it gives you permission to say no to requests that come in. You block off time for meetings at work and things your family needs, but so often you treat your own time as something that can be pushed out or cancelled completely so you can help someone else. Lock in that time for exercise, rest or a treat for yourself and make it immovable. Remember too that no is a complete sentence. You do not have to give big, long, convoluted reasons why you can't do something, as more often than not you'll talk yourself into helping when you're halfway through the sentence. Just say no, I'm sorry I can't, or no, I'm sorry, I have an appointment – nobody needs to know that that appointment is with yourself.

I am in no way saying that you shouldn't give your time to others; of course you should, family and community are very important. You just shouldn't give it to others at the expense of your own happiness or well-being.

Things to say when you want to say no

Q: I know it's late, but could you just finish that document tonight?
Old answer: Em, sure, I'll log back on at home.
New answer: I can't this evening, but I'll do it first thing as a priority.

Q: We're stuck for help again at the club; I know you did it last time but would you mind stepping in?
Old answer: Oh, well, I had plans but if there's no one else, I suppose I could.
New answer: That's so frustrating, I have plans so I can't.

Q: You'll host again, won't you? You're so good at big gatherings.
Old answer: Of course, sure it's no work.
New answer: Let's make a rota so everyone takes a turn.

CASE HISTORY: CARMEL

Carmel came to see me when she was exhausted. She was working three days a week and minding her grandchildren on the other two days. As if that wasn't enough to tire her out, her daughter and her partner were living with her and not helping. Carmel was cooking for them, tidying up after them and doing their washing. They weren't even going to the shops.

Carmel had an autoimmune condition which stemmed from being so run-down. I had a very serious conversation with her about boundaries. She had to learn to sit down and put her feet up. Her daughter and her partner were young adults, well able to do everything for themselves; if they want her to mind their children, they can do everything else in the house or pay for a cleaner.

I see a lot of women of Carmel's generation who do too much and are not empowered enough to say no, enough is enough. She was delighted when I told her to put her feet up – hearing it from a doctor always seems to take the guilt away – but there should be no guilt in having boundaries in the first place. We love our children but we cannot and should not do everything for them. It was clear that Carmel was being taken advantage of and was becoming ill as a result. Boundaries are healthy in every sense of the word.

Recharge and reset

You cannot do everything you want to do if you are mentally and physically exhausted. You will burn out, become hormonally unwell and create a hormonal imbalance. Being all things to all people may seem like you're doing your very best but, in the end, it will come back to haunt you. Recharging and resetting are vital and absolutely related to your boundaries.

Giving yourself time to heal and rest is the greatest gift you can give to yourself and the people around you. Not taking all your allocated holidays, never having a weekend break and not treating yourself doesn't make you the best wife/mother/friend, it makes you a martyr.

Busyness is a disease, it's not a badge of honour. We shouldn't live to work; we should work to live. Take a day off, book a spa break with your friends or go on a weekend away with your partner. If you have young children, get a friend or relative to take them and offer to take theirs in return. Everyone needs a break, everyone needs good-quality rest and everyone needs a laugh!

Mindfulness

At the heart of that time for yourself should be mindfulness. I think a lot of people get confused about what this means and think that they need to meditate or practise some difficult technique, but we can take it back to the very basics.

Take some quiet time for yourself and do something for your mind and your body. You could go for a walk, to a yoga class or sit somewhere you love like the sea or a hilltop and just relax. Don't listen to a podcast or the radio. Don't run through lists in your head of what needs to be done. Just try to clear your mind, take in the view of your surroundings and just be with yourself for a little while.

Breathe deeply, slow down, recharge and reset and make that a priority. Sometimes a bit of mindfulness can just be taking yourself off for a nice coffee on your own, away from the noise at home or the busyness of your work. It doesn't need to be complicated, just restorative.

Positivity

You may, at some stage, have been told to look on the bright side when something bad happened. Someone telling you to cheer up or be positive may be infuriating but there can be a benefit to it. There has been a move in recent years towards positivity as a lifestyle, and while being positive all the time may seem like an unrealistic chore there is a lot to be said for a positive outlook on life.

You don't need to be relentlessly positive – who could manage that with all that's going on in the world? Just adopt a more positive outlook on life. Acknowledge the difficulties but try to put a positive spin on them. Try it on holidays, 'Oh no, it's raining, that's a shame, but hey, what a great day for cosy reading with hot chocolate or board games together.' It becomes easier as you practise.

Positivity also builds resilience, which many people these days find hard to achieve, and helps you to have a more realistic reaction to problems. Resilient people know that there's always an alternative ending, a way to bounce back and a positive outcome to most situations.

A study published in *PNAS* (*Proceedings of the National Academy of Sciences*) in the US in 2019 showed that people with the highest levels of optimism had a longer lifespan (11–15%) on average than those who practised little positive thinking.

We all know positive people in our lives and are mesmerised by how they stay so upbeat even in the face of things going wrong. These people, whether it's a conscious decision or not, are used to being positive and seeing the good in almost every situation. Practice makes perfect and can completely change the way you see the world.

How to practise positivity:

- Tell yourself. It might feel a bit odd at first but picking a personal mantra and repeating it to yourself can help change your outlook when things feel difficult. Choose something like 'I have everything I need' or 'I can get through this' or a mammy favourite like 'What's for you won't pass you'. This can really make you feel better when things are tough.
- Tell yourself a positive story. Instead of always being full of doom and gloom, try to speak positively. If someone at work asks you how your day is going, why not start with the great walk you had at lunchtime or the light traffic on your commute instead of focusing on stress or busyness? How you frame your day in your thoughts will make you think more positively about it.
- Don't suppress your feelings. Of course, bad things do happen and there's no point in trying to cover terrible things with a mask of positivity. Give yourself room to feel your feelings. Grief and sadness need room and time, but remember, your positivity remains in the background for you to return to when you're ready.

- Be grateful. There is a whole industry around gratitude and I'm not saying that you need to go out and invest money in journals or plans. It's enough to start to think regularly about what you're grateful for. Your health, your family, your home, the good weather, your garden, your friends, your job, your holidays – there's a lot to be thankful for and actively remembering them and thinking about some of them each day can make you feel happier and more positive. A study called 'Counting Blessings Versus Burdens: An Experimental Investigation of Gratitude and Subjective Well-Being in Daily Life', published in the *Journal of Personality and Social Psychology* in 2003, asked participants to write a few sentences each week. The cohort was divided into three groups. The first group were asked to write about what they were grateful for, the second were asked to write about things that annoyed them, and the third group were asked to write about the events of the week without any direction towards being positive or negative. The trial lasted for 10 weeks and at the end of it, the researchers found that those who had written about gratitude were happier and more optimistic than the other participants.

It's helpful to remember that everything is a phase, everything is temporary. When things are going well, embrace it, appreciate it, and when things maybe aren't as great, when life is a little more difficult, remember that it doesn't last for ever, that it will change again.

Friendship

As the world changes and people move away from where they were born and raised, friendships grow in importance. While you may see your family a few times a year, friends are the people you see more regularly and with whom you share your life.

It's often said that friends are the family that you choose and anyone with the benefit of close friends knows this to be true. Making friends can be done at any stage in life – it's a myth that it's only for young people. We must keep ourselves active, and finding new hobbies or volunteering in the community are great ways of staying busy, building a local network and finding new friends.

But friendship is not just good for your mind. A study published in the *Journal of Applied Psychology* in 2006 found that loneliness impacts the function of your immune system.

The benefits of friendship have become so important that, according to research done in 2017 by the University of Michigan and published in the journal *Personal Relationships*, having supportive friends is a bigger indicator of well-being than being close to your family.

Of course, in Ireland we've seen the huge work done by the Men's Sheds organisation that has brought men together to form new friendships and build new hobbies. It is an invaluable resource for a group of the population that in the past, once retired, often found themselves lonely.

It's important as we grow older to maintain those special relationships and friendships. Our lives change but isolation and loneliness aren't good for our bodies or minds. Friendships keep us independent, empowered and active.

How to make new friends as an adult

- Join a local group. Most communities have clubs that you can join. You might find fellow readers, a tidy town group or a fundraising committee where you can meet new people with shared interests.
- Say yes to invitations. You never know who you'll meet by going somewhere new. A tablemate at a dinner might become a new friend or a fellow attendee at a local function could be a new companion.
- Don't be afraid to ask. People are all the same and are nervous about making new friends. If you have met someone you think could be a new pal, why don't you ask them for a coffee? If everyone is too nervous to ask, no one will ever make friends!
- Colleagues make wonderful friends. Wouldn't it be terrible to move jobs or retire and never see someone you really like again? Plan some out-of-work meetups so that your friendship is already established away from the office.

Advocate

Being an advocate for yourself is something I feel very passionately about. A huge part of my educational work around menopause and perimenopause is done so that women are armed with enough information to advocate for themselves in medical settings. Doctors are not infallible, remember I say this as one, and you should feel empowered to be firm about your symptoms and getting the treatment you need and to ask questions you want to be answered.

For years in Ireland, we took the word of doctors, priests and anyone with even a modicum of power as gospel. But as we all know now, everyone is human, no one person has all the answers and if something involves you, you have as much right to ask questions as anyone else.

There are things you can do to enable you to become an effective self-advocate:

1 **Believe in yourself.** You can only effectively advocate for yourself when you have the confidence to know that you're as good as the people you're dealing with.
2 **Educate yourself.** Read as much as you can about whatever situation you find yourself in, whether it's medical, legal or work-related.
3 **Know what you want.** Have a clear plan and end goal in place.
4 **Express yourself.** Asking questions and pushing for the resolution you want can be daunting. Stay calm, speak clearly and bring notes so that you don't forget any questions or important points you want to make.
5 **Be firm.** Don't be fobbed off, don't give up. When people know that you're persistent and confident they will be more likely to take you seriously.

Women have often been accused of being emotional or angry in a way that men asking questions never are, but that was always just a way to stop women from speaking up and self-advocating. Thankfully, things have changed a lot, but I still hear of women being afraid to ask questions of their doctors and surgeons, so

I want to be clear: never be afraid to ask a question about your health. Women know their bodies better than anyone and if you feel something is wrong or there is a question to be asked about your care, you should ask it. Be empowered to speak up, speak loudly and get answers.

How to ask questions at a doctor's appointment

- Write down all the concerns you would like to have addressed and list them in order of importance.
- Know what your desired outcome is, whether that's further tests, a referral to a consultant or medication.
- Have a list of symptoms and dates that you can refer back to.
- If you feel you aren't being listened to, repeat your concerns and outline what you would like to happen.
- If you feel unsatisfied and your GP practice has more than one doctor, see if you can make an appointment with someone else.
- Remember that you and your GP should have a relationship of trust. If you don't feel you're getting that or what you need, you're entitled to change GP.

Comparison is the thief of rest

There is an external factor that weighs heavily on our ability to rest. Social media has become an all-pervasive force and one which many of us find hard to ignore or tune out. It may seem silly or trivial, but if you think about your reaction to what you see on Instagram or ask your friends or family about it you will soon discover how powerful a factor it is.

Many of us spend hours on social media these days and while in the past you may have heard people talking about 'keeping up with the Joneses', we are now trying to keep up with people we only know by watching them on a tiny screen.

It does everything from making us want to buy more and more clothes to feeling bad about the state of our homes because a stranger on the internet always has a perfectly gleaming kitchen.

It sounds bizarre when you break it down like this, but it is an insidious beast built to draw us in and keep us addicted. You finish a day's work and sit down for an hour to relax and find yourself picking up your phone and scrolling and scrolling through perfect houses, beautiful ageless faces and immaculate wardrobes. But remember that you never see the row that woman has had with her partner, or how lonely the girl with the gorgeous coat is, or the nanny or the cleaner, or the doctor with a Botox needle. Social media is a highlight reel, it is the best parts of the day that people choose to share, not every part of the day.

If you feel bad for cooking oven chips because someone you follow cooks from scratch every night or think that your sink should be shining before you get into bed, remember that what you are seeing is not real.

We know that women are all too prone to thinking that we should be doing it all and having it all the way that men do, but you can only do so much. Remember that a lot of those very successful men who do it all often have a partner at home doing the cooking, washing and planning.

If you wonder why our politicians have never been that interested in providing proper subsidised childcare, remember that it is because most of them are men with partners who looked after all of that. They're not interested because it has never been an issue for them. Imagine the luxury of not having to think about who is minding your children.

Children are another area of comparison I see a lot. Thinking that your child is falling behind because they're not doing eight activities a week, having grinds in every subject and doing every summer camp available will quickly have you feeling exhausted from the logistics of it all and poor from the cost. Children need your love and attention and whatever else you can give them is a bonus. Because one woman at school or a stranger on Instagram has her children scheduled to within an inch of their lives is not a reason for you to do it and it doesn't make it right.

Comparison is causing burnout. Getting up at 6 a.m. to work out is depriving you of rest. Influencers get sent a lot of free clothes; you should not and could not keep up with that. Everyone's home is untidy sometimes; children need to feel bored – it's good for them; a frozen pizza never killed anyone and those women on your phone aren't showing you everything.

Social media can be great – I use it all the time to share information and show what I'm doing with my work. It's when it's starting to make you feel bad that you should put it down. Read a book, watch TV or listen to a podcast in the evenings instead. You don't need to polish the inside of your sink because a stranger on the internet does.

Carpe diem

If you follow me on social media you may have heard me say carpe diem – seize the day – quite a lot. I am so aware that as my children grow – my twin boys are 18 years old now – time moves incredibly quickly. The global pandemic taught us so much about what is important in our lives and how fragile life is. I know my children won't always be able, or want, to come on holiday with me. I'm excited to see them grow and live their own wonderful lives but I want to enjoy every moment of them now while I can. We're all so busy, young and old, so if I see an opportunity to get away with my family, I grab it. I said before about how important holidays were for the four of us after my husband passed away and they continue to be a wonderful way for us all to bond and spend time together.

I carpe diem by taking breaks away, spending time with my wonderful extended family and seeing my friends, but for you it might be a work opportunity, a night out with friends, the chance to have a break with your partner or just some time for yourself. What's important is that we seize the day and welcome these things with open arms. We have but one life and we should do everything in our power to enjoy it as much as we possibly can. You'll always be more disappointed in the things you didn't do than the things you did do. I think you'd be hard-pushed to find anyone on their deathbed who wishes they'd taken fewer holidays with their loved ones or said no to more opportunities to laugh and enjoy themselves. Sure if you didn't laugh you'd cry – this is a wonderful Irish saying and I love to see people have fun living their wonderful lives.

Change is needed

If we are serious about empowering society, we must become more equal as a society and empower our young girls to be equal to our boys. If we do that, they will have high self-esteem and self-worth and will understand how to have effective boundaries in life and work. It starts in childhood, earlier than you think, and we must do everything we can to show our children how clever and fantastic they are.

If we look around us we can see there's still a lot of work to be done. Great, positive strides have been made in sport to level the playing field with opportunities for women, equal pay for teams and equal coverage of men's and women's sport on national TV, but there is still more to do.

We must work hard to have women in visible roles in politics and business, to get rid of the gender pay gap, to achieve parity in gender roles and childcare, and in religion.

I want to see lots of female CEOs, a female Taoiseach and female priests. I want our women front and centre. I want us to truly see equality. Women are 50% of our society, after all. I want to see women also not being afraid to challenge tradition and to be seen doing so. I was recently at a wedding where the groom, groom's father and best man spoke and neither the bride nor any of her bridesmaids gave a speech. Women must see it as their role to be seen to be equal. There is no point in some of us trying our best to achieve gender equality if all women are not coming on board to make sure that this is the case and even if they only say two words they are at least showing that they are equal and deserve to be heard too.

For too long we have allowed this total inequality to go on without questioning how destructive it is to our society. We are so busy that it can be hard to see what we can do, but there is a lot. We can vote for women, give women-owned businesses our money, we can speak up where we see inequality and unfairness and we can demand the very necessary change that needs to happen in all areas of our society.

We need more positive female voices talking about women's health, hormones and menopause because without that nothing changes, and if nothing changes nothing will ever change.

CASE HISTORY: MICHELLE

I met Michelle during the Covid lockdowns. She came to me with a severe hormonal imbalance. We sat together and talked through what was going on in her life. I quickly discovered that Michelle's mother was calling on her to do everything from collecting her shopping to getting prescriptions. This would be fine, only Michelle lived 15km from her mother and had two brothers who lived beside her but who were never called upon at all.

I asked why this was happening and she told me that her mother thought that the 'boys' were too busy and that it was Michelle's job.

The problem here was that Michelle's mother was unconsciously putting her sons on a pedestal and abusing her daughter's kindness. The same had probably been done to her and this is where we see the old cycles perpetuated. Young men are not busier than young women and it is not automatically a woman's job to look after older parents. Where there are siblings, this job has to be a shared one. Michelle's mother was unconsciously contributing to her daughter's low self-esteem as she had high expectations of her but not of her sons.

I asked Michelle to stop doing it all alone and to speak to her brothers. I also asked her how she would feel if in 20 years' time she saw her daughter doing the same thing for her mother-in-law.

Her brothers should have stepped in and offered to help, but if a family dynamic is set up like this the people who don't have to do the extra work are often happy to let the status quo lie. Think about what you would say to your daughter or your friends if you saw them in a situation like this and then say those words to yourself.

Michelle stopped doing it all and after some rest, treatment and changes to her lifestyle, she got back to full health.

Final words

I hope that this book has helped you see the importance of hormones in your life and understand what endocrinology is. Hormones are our body's control centre and are responsible for more functions than you could ever imagine.

Hormones control our entire world.

They control our muscles, our immune system, our emotions, our sex, whether we are male or female, our ability to fall in love, our smell, our need to eat, our need to survive, our sense of danger.

They are behind our ability to procreate, our desire to procreate, our ability to enjoy, to feel stressed, to sleep, to stay awake and to dream.

In order for hormones to be balanced there is a lot we can do to help ourselves. Eating healthily, getting adequate sleep and having a good work–life balance are the first steps in taking control of our hormonal health.

The most important thing we need to have a healthy hormone system is high self-esteem and a high sense of self-worth. We need to love ourselves enough to take care of ourselves properly and make self-care a priority.

Our society has never been great at telling women that they are important or that they matter. Things are changing, but those changes can feel incredibly slow. By working together, we are a powerful machine of change that will make life better for the young women growing up now. Women must not be afraid to act as mentors and change traditional narratives. A lot of my female patients feel cheated when, after nine months of pregnancy, society expects their child to only use their husband's surname. It's important that women feel empowered to deviate from this tradition. I kept my own name when I married and my children have double-barrelled surnames. There's no reason why a woman shouldn't feel empowered to do this if it's what she wants.

So much has been done, but we need more. We need more research into hormonal health and women's health in particular, which up to recently has been seriously lacking.

We need more research into endometriosis and the effect of heavy periods on the hormonal system as well as long-term studies into the safety of the oral contraceptive pill over a long period as girls are now becoming sexualised so young. We also need more research into PCOS and infertility in men and women.

We need to improve education in schools and with the public around periods, perimenopause, menopause, contraception, vasectomy, equal responsibility of the sexes for contraception and postmenopause health in women. We need to educate boys and girls equally.

We need more support for women after childbirth and a better understanding of menstrual problems and support structures for the women in our society who are suffering.

We need more research into women's heart disease post-menopause, osteoporosis and the higher incidence of autoimmune disease in women and what we can do to prevent it.

And we really need to do more to achieve equality of the sexes so that women have support and options.

Tips for good hormonal health

- Empowerment of self. Remember, we all have a great power within us but need to realise it and see it. We do not need any external person to validate us – we have ourselves. Have self-love and believe in yourself. This self-love will keep your hormonal vortex and balance in tune and it will empower you and your overall health.
- Healthy eating and nourishment
- Appropriate sleep
- Appropriate relaxation
- Meditation
- Regular check-ups with your doctor regarding your hormonal and overall health – and listen to the advice.

My wish for you through this book is for you to understand the impact that minding yourself has on hormonal health and how looking after yourself, being equal in your home and enjoying your life, friends and family can improve your overall health.

Life is wonderful, ageing is a privilege, and being a woman is a great gift.

Let's enjoy every part of it.

Acknowledgements

Thank you to Sarah Liddy, Jennifer Stevens and Margaret Farrelly from Gill Books and all the wonderful people who made this dream possible.

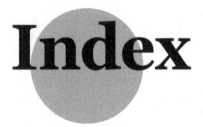

Index

Index